BOOBS
ARE
OVERRATED

Breast
Reconstruction,
Cancer Scars, and the
Unfiltered Truth

CAROL WYLLIE

Published by: DubPress
Cover Design:
Copyright © 2024 by Carol Wyllie

Boobs Are Overrated

Although the author and publisher have made every effort to ensure that the information in this book was correct at press time, the author and publisher do not assume and hereby disclaim any liability to any party for any loss, damage, or disruption caused by errors or omissions, whether such errors or omissions result from negligence, accident, or any other cause.

Adherence to all applicable laws and regulations, including international, federal, state and local governing professional licensing, business practices, advertising, and all other aspects of doing business in the US, Canada or any other jurisdiction is the sole responsibility of the reader and consumer.

Neither the author nor the publisher assumes any responsibility or liability whatsoever on behalf of the consumer or reader of this material. Any perceived slight of any individual or organization is purely unintentional.

The resources in this book are provided for informational purposes only and should not be used to replace the specialized training and professional judgment of a health care or mental health care professional. The book is not intended to be a substitute for professional medical advice, diagnosis or treatment.

Neither the author nor the publisher can be held responsible for the use of the information provided within this book. Please always consult a qualified and/or licensed physician or other medical care provider before making any decision regarding treatment of yourself or others.

ISBN: 978-1-959583-05-9 Paperback
ISBN: 978-1-959583-06-6 Ebook

Thank you for purchasing my book.
Please enjoy this free gift as a token of my appreciation:
Visit https://www.wylliegirl.com to download
your Cheat Sheet and bonus chapter.

Dedication

To my husband, Rob, and all the caregivers out there.
Even though you didn't get cancer and
treatment and surgeries, you did.

Table of Contents

Introduction

My stomach dropped. My pits began to sweat. Every nerve ending went on high alert as my skin tingled. Like when you almost get into a car accident and your system floods with adrenaline right after the near miss. Or that first second at the top of a roller coaster when you start to drop. Except I was in a dark room of the hospital, hearing the words I'd come to dread. Not a pitch black room for sleeping, but it was muted. Maybe for some calming effect, or just so they could see their screens better.

Lying on my left side, with a foam wedge underneath my right side and my back to the door, I felt anything but calm—even before the bottom dropped out of my day. I heard the door open and craned my neck a little to see the radiologist walk in, followed by the tech who just finished my ultrasound. The doctor was a small, quirky looking man I remembered from the previous routine scan I'd had, probably a year prior. He greeted me generically so I knew he didn't remember me, nor did I expect him to. He began his own ultrasound and clinically explained what he did as he went along, pointing out images on the screen. The screen was completely behind me and above my head. The angle made it hard to see, even if I could decipher the shadows and images. But I just went with it as un-awkwardly as possible.

"I think we should do a biopsy," he said. My ears began ringing. I exhaled a breath I didn't realize I was holding. "See all these little Oreos? Those are your lymph nodes."

I still didn't see anything except a bunch of weird lines and shadows. But I nodded and continued to crane my neck to follow his finger and tutorial.

"See this one lymph node right here?" I didn't really, but I nodded. "The one that looks different?"

I nodded again. I couldn't make words. What would I have said, anyway?

"With your history, I'd recommend a biopsy. Just to be cautious. It's probably benign."

I nodded again, but it felt like slow motion. I asked if this weird lymph node could be from a recent bout of food poisoning I'd had. I saw the nurse smile like she would at a small child who said something ridiculous, just as the doctor began to shake his head.

"No, it doesn't work that way."

I always thought swollen lymph nodes were a sign of infection. You know how we can feel swollen glands when we're sick? Like that. Apparently, that wasn't what he was seeing. *This can't be happening again.* He did say it was most likely benign, but he wanted to be cautious. *Thank you for that.* But this wasn't my first rodeo. *Didn't they all say that initially?* I think it's something they say to try to keep us calm while we wait for tests and scans and results.

The nurse led me to the dressing room where I got dressed, then headed to the scheduler to make the biopsy appointment. She gave me the first available one which was two weeks away. Two weeks of talking myself off the ledge and mentally chanting his words, "likely benign." The scheduler did say she always gets cancellations and would most likely be calling me if I were open for last minute appointments. I assured her I'd be available. She called within two days to schedule me for a Sunday biopsy. Yep! A Sunday! Who knew they even did procedures on a Sunday? Not me. But I jumped on it. Just four days of internal chanting versus two weeks.

I mentioned to the scheduler that I saw in the paperwork they would be doing a "gentle" mammogram after the biopsy to verify that the biopsy marker was in place. I let her know there couldn't be any mammogram happening to my very newly constructed live tissue breast, gentle or otherwise, and gave her a quick rundown of my surgical history. She made *ooh* and *ahh* sounds and took copious notes and even asked how to spell "omentum" so she got it right for the doctor. She assured me all of that info would be in my chart and the doctor would see it.

In case you're wondering about my internal dialogue, it went something like this:

> *God, please let it be nothing. I've just been given my clean bill of health. I'm finally getting to live my life with some semblance of normalcy. Please God. I want to grow old with my husband, see my children get married and have their own kids, and be healthy. Just breathe,*

Carol. You're healed. You're healthy. You're well. In Jesus' name. It's nothing. NOTHING!

Along with the internal dialogue, I was trying *not* to envision my family's life without me. It was dark, and paralyzing. And usually hit me at night when it was quiet and there were no distractions. My go-to was reading. I highly recommend a good plot. One that can transport you to another world where your thoughts are drowned out by fictional characters. Music was another sure tool for transporting me out of my current world and my head. Nothing can take me to a specific point in time like a song lyric. And it became my go-to over the next few days of waiting and overthinking, whenever I found myself in my car. Driving home that day after the ultrasound, I blared 80s hair band rock music so loud in my car that it hurt my ears, but in a good way. The angrier the song, the better.

On the day of the biopsy, my past biopsy results played in my head on a loop, closely followed by my internal chants. I waded through my pool of coping methods for four days and the drive to the hospital was my deep end. I did yoga breathing like it was my lifeline. And wasn't it? God bless my husband. He had his own chant. When he heard my chain of deep breaths, he squeezed my hand and said, "It's nothing."

The cool thing about Sunday procedures is the place is quiet—calm, even. I tried not to study the face of the nurse who called me back and escorted me to the dark room; at the last *bad news* biopsy appointment, many years ago, I could tell by the look on the nurse's face before the doctor said a word. This wasn't going to be a results appointment, anyway, but the procedure itself had me worked up. Biopsies were painful and, frankly, barbaric. My body had been through enough. That was my new chant as I waited for the radiologist to come in.

This was a different radiologist than the one who talked about Oreos and *wanted* the biopsy. She was tiny, friendly, and articulate. She came in, leaned against the counter, and began telling me that with my history, she felt confident it was nothing. *OH MY GOD. Say more!* She did!

"You are only three months out of a major surgery?" I nodded. "Yeah, your body is still healing. I would rather not further traumatize the area with a biopsy, because chances are what we're seeing is the lymph nodes reacting to that state of healing. I'm going to do another ultrasound right now just to confirm that, but I feel pretty certain that's what's happening."

Oh. Em. Gee. So she is basing this on the information I gave the scheduler. Thank God I told the scheduler! What if I hadn't? Why can't these frickin' teaching hospitals share information?

Sidebar: my surgeries took place at a different teaching hospital than the one doing my scans. I'd been a patient at all three renowned teaching hospitals in my area. The first one for chemo, because that is where I found the biggest, baddest rockstar doctor for breast cancer. Once it was time for my daily radiation, the radiologist from that hospital said he could not, in good conscience, suggest driving to him everyday for treatment.

"You run a higher risk of a car accident than a recurrence," he'd said.

He called a medical school colleague at another teaching hospital just an hour away from me to get me set up there for radiation. Eventually, that hospital referred me to yet another one for the reconstruction. Once upon a time, they all shared information via the patient online portals. Apparently—according to one employee I spoke to at some point over the years—they stopped sharing information. I never got the reason. I just know it adds another unnecessary layer to patient advocacy. And yes, I'd signed all the forms so each of them could obtain any records they wanted. But they had to know they wanted or needed them to request them.

This doctor positioned me like before—my back to her, lying half on a wedge, arm over my head, neck craned toward her and the machine. Right away she said that she didn't even think the lymph node in question was *one* lymph node, but two on top of each other appearing as one abnormal one. Her professional opinion was to recheck me in six to eight weeks, after more healing had taken place. Every single cell in my body seemed to exhale at once. I think I floated back to the dressing room. Once I closed that curtain, I almost hit my knees. I began chanting internally, *Thank you, Jesus! Thank you, Jesus! Thank you, Jesus!*

When I walked out into the waiting room just minutes after going in, my husband looked at me questioningly.

"It's nothing," I said. "Let's get out here."

I almost ran out of that place. Or levitated. I walk fast normally anyway, but I took it to a whole new level that day. I felt euphoric. I wanted to celebrate. So did he. If we needed a reminder to live in the moment and take nothing for granted, mission accomplished.

I wish I could say that the anxiety associated with cancer and scans and pretty much every ache, pain, or malady goes away. I'm hopeful, but so far, it hasn't. I tell myself it's a good reminder to count my blessings. And—not to go too country song on you here, but maybe it helps us forgive more readily, give the benefit of the doubt more often, and cross more things off our bucket lists. Maybe it just allows us to trust that we've finally come to the end of our struggle tunnel and we can trust that the light we see is the dawn of a new day and not a train. But when the last two years of my life were seemingly one reconstruction train after another, I readily understood my hesitation.

Chapter 1

Hindsight Is 20/20

For those who haven't read my first book, *Chemo Pissed Me Off*, here's a little background—the condensed version:

I wasn't supposed to get cancer. I know—is anyone *supposed to* get cancer? What I mean is that I was in no high-risk categories. I had no genetic markers or family history, I wasn't overweight, nor was I a smoker. I wish I had a dollar for every time a doctor told me my cancer was just bad luck. Nothing sets me off quite like that. *Seriously?! Bad luck?* All that medical school, student loans, missed sleep, and the best you've got is "bad luck?" I don't even have words for this ridiculousness. And as a writer, I pretty much always have words.

I also don't believe "everything happens for a reason." I know, unpopular opinion. And maybe I didn't always believe that. I know for sure I've poetically proclaimed "everything happens for a reason" plenty of times, in some ill attempt at inspiration or compassion. But did I truly believe it, or did I just say it because it seemed like the thing to say at the moment? Probably the latter, if I'm being honest. My go-to line for things people say without the critical thinking behind it to back it up is "just make it make sense." So, on my quest to *make it make sense*, I realized that for me, it just didn't.

Follow me down my rabbit hole for a moment.

I believe in God and the power of prayer. I believe in the Bible, although I think it is largely taken out of context by fallible, imperfect humans so we can make sense of the fallen world we live in.

I believe that bad things happen because of our fallen world of imperfect humans and our free will of choice. We are driven by ego, immaturity, and selfishness; sometimes, we make bad decisions which, as a result, lead to bad consequences and ripple effects we could never even fathom. I hear you fellow critical thinkers asking if I then believe cancer is the result of someone's bad choice. The short answer is: *possibly*, in some convoluted, roundabout way. The longer answer is most likely a whole other book that I do not have the authority nor expertise to even attempt to write. So I'll stay in my lane. But (... yes, there is a but):

> In Romans 8:28 we read, "And we know that in all things God works for the good of those who love him, who have been called according to his purpose." (NIV)

My *mere mortal* interpretation of this scripture is that while bad things may happen (i.e. breast cancer, horrific treatments, and nightmare reconstruction surgeries), God can and will use those things for our ultimate good—if we love him, and if we believe. Before

I lose you on the assumption that this is some preachy book, hear me out. One of my favorite Christian authors and thought leaders, Norman Vincent Peale, notably had two best friends, each of a different spiritual background. He said the important thing was to *have* a spiritual belief—a belief in something bigger than ourselves. To keep us grounded, humble, seeking, and growing. Maybe it's the law of attraction for you—that's one of my favorites, and I personally believe it exists as tangibly as gravity. Or karma—the Biblical equivalent is "reaping what you sow." Whatever label you choose to put on it, I believe that God prepares us for things if we pay attention and may even teach us something in the midst.

I do not believe that there is some predestined plan that some of us will get cancer and fight for our lives. And to that end, I am *not* grateful I got cancer. Cancer is bullshit! But I do believe God took this shitty situation and used it to teach me a few things, adjust my perspective, enrich my life, and bring me the desires of my heart (Psalms 37:4)—like realizing my lifelong dream of becoming a self-published, bestselling author. And it started with my breast cancer diagnosis about thirteen years ago. While I'm beyond grateful to have realized my dream, I might be more specific in praying for the vehicle that takes me there in the future. So, maybe I am grateful for cancer in some roundabout way, yet it's too awful for me to wholeheartedly give it any credit. I'd rather believe God took the cancer and found a detour to the good stuff.

We've all heard the saying, "Hindsight is 20/20." I believe it! It's true, if we pay attention. At the age of forty-one, I was diagnosed with breast cancer(ish).

It was technically pre-cancer, called ductal carcinoma in situ (DCIS). Throughout this ordeal, I've heard repeatedly how well I've handled it all. I did not wake up one day and decide to be good at cancer, but I paid attention. And I believe without a doubt that God prepared me for it; thankfully, he began doing so well before my diagnosis.

My *preparation* began, weirdly enough, in a Walmart. Proof that God has a sense of humor? I think so. Almost exactly one year before my diagnosis, we visited Elko, Nevada for my husband's family reunion, as we did almost every July until his father's passing. I was browsing through the book section—because thirteen years ago, when you found yourself in Elko, Walmart is what you *did*—when I found a book I'd been meaning to read: *90 Minutes in Heaven* by Don Piper. I was in vacation mode, and it seemed like a good time to read it. My two biggest takeaways from the book were the power of prayer and how badly I wanted to hear God—really *hear* God—when he spoke to me.

In my quest to hear God, after we returned home from vacation, I joined a new Bible study at my church. This in and of itself was big for me. I was not a joiner and I could regularly be heard saying that not all of us are called to big, philanthropic acts of faith—some of us are called to take up space in the pews on Sundays. But I eagerly joined. It was called Rock Solid and was all about hearing the voice of God. Check! And it was a big commitment of joining—twenty-six weeks long! Still, I jumped in with both feet.

A month or so into the study, I found myself on the scene of a horrific car accident in my rural town of roughly 10,000 people. A few months after that, I ended up on the scene of another accident in my small town. I started feeling like The Accident Girl. I also felt like God had called me to those accidents to be with the two women victims in their time of need. Like I was hearing God tell me I needed to be available in times of need. I was grateful He had called me and that I'd heard Him.

In the first accident, a woman was riding a motorcycle and was struck by a truck. She was screaming in pain and crying hysterically, lying on the pavement, essentially bleeding out. At one point, her breathing got shallow and I knew without knowing that it wasn't a good sign. I began praying over her, holding her hand and petting her face to keep her calm until the emergency personnel arrived. She nearly lost her life, but instead only lost her leg.

In the second accident, it was a rainy morning—a woman lost control of her car and hit an oncoming vehicle. Without a thought—except maybe subconsciously saying to myself, *here we go again*—I hopped out of my car and rushed to the driver's side window of the unconscious woman. I climbed down into a muddy ditch in the rain to get to her. I held her hand and began talking to her and praying for her. I later found out that the woman didn't make it. Both experiences were traumatic and haunting, but I was convinced I was hearing God and genuinely grateful He was using me to help others.

A few months later, while on our yearly vacation again in Elko, I'd heard through the small town grapevine that the motorcycle woman wanted to meet the woman who prayed for her and stayed with her. I planned to meet her when I got home. Instead, I got diagnosed with breast cancer(ish).

I say "ish" because some people don't think DCIS *is* cancer. But when there is something in your body that wants to take over and try to kill you, I think you can call it what you want. I didn't care what they called it—I wanted it gone. I was only forty-one. My children were young and they needed their mom. Right away I wanted a mastectomy, and even wanted the healthy one removed for peace of mind. I instantly replied, "Take them." It hit me then, the detours God can and does take to bring us to the good stuff. While God may have very well sent me to those women, he also sent them to me to show me that this ordeal I would face—the mastectomy, for starters—was not a leg, and it was not my life. It was just boobs. And I could do this!

Do I believe these women were meant to get into accidents to show me some perspective? Abso-fucking-lutely not! But I believe God can take the *fucked up-ness* of this life and use it for something good. For me, this is way more palatable than some predetermined fate or, worse, a roll of the dice. I'd like to believe we have some control over our lives or at least a good takeaway when things don't go our way. Speaking of things not going my way, breast reconstruction is a years-long process. It is a marathon, not a sprint—and speaking of running, I never did understand the Zen of running. Much like this boob marathon. I'm not sure I understand the what, why, or how of it all, even today. Now that I'm on the other side of it, I'm still not sure I could successfully sell it to someone else. It is one hell of a commitment to boobs. Am I happy to be done? Oh yeah. Am I happy to have boobs? For sure. Are boobs overrated? I'm leaning that way, but I'll let you be the judge.

Chapter 2

How'd We Get Here?

A re boobs overrated?
    The short answer: opinions vary.

My long(er) answer:
Perhaps.

From my induction into the Itty Bitty Titty Committee at puberty and my yearly membership renewal throughout my teens and twenties, younger me would vote that they are overrated. When attempting to breastfeed my two children, I'd venture to say all three of us might've agreed at one point that my boobs were overrated. The eldest took forever to find her latch, but eventually figured it out—with a lot of fussing and crying (from me, not her). My second had a perfect latch and we gelled from the jump, but she was violently *allergic* to my milk. It became an issue of nourishment over the breastfeeding supermom medal of honor. And, PSA for any new moms and moms-to-be out there: don't let anyone shame you into breastfeeding. While it is absolutely my first choice, if it's not working, it's not working. There is no award for breastfeeding. We are all different. I wish I'd known and believed this with the birth of my first child, who was so colicky, distended, and miserable. I for sure wish I'd known this when every nurse and doctor I encountered pressured me to jump through ridiculous hoops to breastfeed from the moment I became a mom.

At forty-one, when diagnosed with DCIS and opting for a double mastectomy, I would concur: overrated. I was a young stay-at-home mom with young kids, and my boobs were apparently trying to kill me ... at least, the left one was. So yeah, I was over my boobs and I needed to get back to my life and the kids who needed me in it. I opted for the quick-fix of implants, since my mastectomies negated the need for further treatment. Implant surgeries were outpatient with minimal recovery time. Also, after implants, I got to turn in my card for the Itty Bitty Titty Committee and became Barbie instead—perfectly sized, perky breasts ... sans nipples.

And remember, I wasn't in any high-risk categories, so I wasn't even supposed to get cancer. I guess someone forgot to tell my boobs that. My incessant curiosity and need to *make it make sense* would set in motion a rabbit hole of deep dives into whole-body health that has spanned thirteen years and counting.

At forty-nine, when a small amount of breast tissue left behind in my axilla (underarm area) grew from DCIS to invasive ductal carcinoma (IDC) Stage 1/ Grade 3 and required *all* the toxic cancer treatments, no doubt: overrated. My fifty-first year on earth didn't begin with a festive party celebrating the big five-oh, nor that tropical vacation we'd planned. It began instead with four rounds of chemo for cancer I no longer had, followed by a month of radiation, all because of a bit of breast tissue a surgeon left behind eight years prior. When the doctor told me the news, I asked how I could possibly have breast cancer without any boobs. He said some medical stuff about recurrences, but the one comment that stood out to me was this: "Eight years is a long time."

FOR WHOM?!

Granted, my kids were almost adults and didn't need me as much anymore, but I wasn't ready to give up my residency on the planet. And the surgery itself got *all* the cancer, so I was pissed I even had to have toxic treatments. They were an insurance policy, they said, in case any microscopic cancer cells were left behind. That's a hefty, toxic, disgusting insurance policy. Don't get me started on that. We'll just put that in the box labeled "All the stupid shit doctors say."

At fifty-two, I needed to remove my implants due to contracture damage from surgery, a subsequent seroma, followed by a month of radiation. To calm my immune system down and help prevent a recurrence, I opted to undergo a fourteen-hour DIEP flap surgery (deep inferior epigastric perforator) to make live tissue breasts. After this, I'd vote hell yes: overrated, especially after one of those flaps died and required an emergency surgery ten days later to remove the dead tissue and stop the bleeding. This was when I began to wonder what the hell I was doing all that for. Boobs? Obviously, yes. But the answer is a little more nuanced than that.

At fifty-three, eleven months after that surgery and still waiting for a corrective surgery while sporting one live tissue breast and one concave ... area where a breast should be, absolutely: *overrated!* Suffice it to say, it wasn't a good look. Thankfully, Billie Eilish, in all her *iconic-ness*, made the "extreme baggy shirt" look a fashion statement around this time. No, I didn't look at all like an older mom trying to be a cool mom and dress like a kid. I might've preferred that to what I saw in the mirror: a baggy mom possibly over caring about her appearance. I assure you, that's not me. I like to dress the part and shamelessly match whenever possible, and it's always possible. I learned early on in my ordeal not to wear things I actually liked or carry favorite bags with favorite socks or blankets. It's strange how certain things have a "cancer ick factor" now by association, like outfits worn to and from the hospital. I'd collected some clothing I couldn't even look at, let alone wear anymore because of their ties to some of my darkest days. I highly recommend special *cancer stuff* that can go away with the treatment—like the baggy shirts, which I donated to a thrift store afterward.

Though my family and friends repeatedly told me otherwise (they're good like that), I embodied a frumpy, middle-aged woman who might've lost her fashion sense. I was also knee-deep in navigating the "cancer hair grow out" phase. I'll just say it: I had a mullet! And not by choice. I wasn't trying to resurrect a trend that shouldn't have been born to begin with. I used *the cold cap* during chemo to try to keep my hair—unlike some women, who treated the bald head thing like a badge of honor. Losing my hair might've scared me more than (or at least as much as) chemo did. And a quick rundown on cold caps: they work by cooling the scalp, temporarily constricting blood flow to your hair follicles. This reduces the amount of drug (chemo) that reaches your hair, as well as the metabolic activity of your follicles, making them less sensitive to chemo's effects. It boasts that it can usually guarantee you keep about 50 percent of your hair. I have a lot of hair, so I envisioned having thin hair for a bit. And because I didn't *have* cancer, it became weirdly important to me that I didn't *look* like I had cancer.

Fun fact about cold caps is they don't factor in which 50 percent would give the best aesthetics. I lost my 50 percent on the top of my head. I looked like an 80s rocker hanging onto my glory days. Technically, I was considered a cold cap success. I didn't hold my breath waiting to be their poster child. Needless to say, it was not a good look. In the spirit of staying positive, though, I was digging deep to find my silver linings, and I dug like it was my job. There were so many reminders of the shitty side of all this that it became my mission to take back my life.

Thanks to a ridiculous pandemic, I mostly isolated that year waiting for the "fix-it" surgery to ensure I was healthy. I was ready to go if I got greenlit to fill a last-minute cancellation, but no such luck. What I did get was repeated cancellations to my own surgery date. Yeah, I'd say it's official: I'm firmly in the camp of boobs being overrated—and maybe a little more than slightly in the camp of thinking the whole cancer medical world sucks. But I can say that the pandemic gave me a great excuse to hide my mullet and my boob hole as much as possible. See me digging deep? Because cancer can no doubt throw some curveballs of utter crap at us, we take our celebrations where we can get them. It's what we do with the curveballs of crap that counts. Finding our silver linings in the crap is when the magic happens. But first, the crap ...

My *crap* looked like over seventy-five visits to a teaching hospital an hour away, sometimes daily over a period of four years; over sixty-five visits to another teaching hospital two to three hours away, depending which office I went to; three major surgeries; one outpatient surgery; over ten visits to a concierge-certified lymphedema therapist two-and-a-half hours away (which, incidentally, wasn't covered by insurance); many failed attempts at purchasing lymphedema garments and far fewer failed attempts to find a reliable therapist to help me navigate it all (without, you know, becoming a complete asshole to everyone around me in the frustration and juggling of it all). For those doing the math, that's over 150 separate medical-related incidents. I told you, it was like a full-time job—except I wasn't getting paid. In fact, I was the one paying—and not just in money.

I know! I can hear you already:

> *Why did she do it? I'd have said, "Screw that." So not worth it. And who has time or money for all that? That is a stupid level of commitment to boobs.*

First, I hear you! Second, let me explain.

Chapter 3

I Just Want Boobs

"Desire is the key to motivation,
but it's determination and commitment to an
unrelenting pursuit of your goal – a commitment to
excellence –
that will enable you to attain the success you seek.
~Mario Andretti

I'm just going to say it. I still wanted boobs, for a lot of reasons. Cancer takes so much and leaves a trail of destruction in its wake—chemo fatigue and brain fog, radiation tattoos, burns and discoloration, surgery scars and deformities, and too many body aches to count, just to name a few. I guess I wanted to take my life back, undo some of the damage cancer had done, and emerge a better version of myself. I wanted to prove to myself and others that cancer did not win, that there is always hope. Cheesy *woo woo-ness* aside, I believe that with every fiber of my being.

The easiest reason might be so that I could stop overthinking my outfits every frickin' time I got dressed, thought about getting dressed, or left my house for any reason. I'm just going to play my girl card here and say that I think about fashion—not in a Kardashian way, but I do. And I know not only girls think about fashion, so no disrespect, guys. I like to look cute, or pretty, or hot, or just appropriately attired for the event at hand. It could be cut-off shorts and an 80s rocker tee (lucky for me, this fashion trend went with my mullet), but I like to be clad for the vibe—whatever that may be. And swimsuits ... ugh! Even those baggy ones, as soon as they're wet, cling to everything. Swimming attire may arguably be the most vulnerable outfit that exists in the chick world. We're hyper-aware of unwanted dimples and cellulite, muffin tops and belly bloat, stretch marks and saggy arms. Can we not add deformed boobs to the list? It's the most naked most of us ever are in public, and I like to dial down the freak show whenever possible.

One of the biggest things for me is to have a body that isn't a constant reminder of the cancer shit show. I mean, in my case, I'll never have real nipples again, but I can have a chest that doesn't scream "CANCER" every frickin' time I look in the mirror, jump in the shower, or change my clothes. And thank you, Barbie, for making no nipples cool. It saved me a surgery/procedure and the pain of more tattoos. Tattooed nipples are a thing in the breast cancer world, in case you didn't know. And I like tattoos, but the last thing I needed or wanted was more procedures. There will always be plenty of scars, but I can almost see past them now, as time goes on. A silhouette that looks like me goes a long way.

For the record, *me* is a subjective term. Younger me was very petite with a chest to match. Pre-cancer, post-childbirth *me* had gravity—and nursing-afflicted "pancake" boobs that mostly got rolled into some kind of bra to contain them. Post-cancer/round one *me* had "store bought" implants that looked like God was just really nice to me. So when I say *me*, what I really mean is a chest that (like I said) isn't a constant reminder of cancer and the shit show I endured. And let's just get this out the way: a chest that *feels* like *me* (mostly, anyway) goes a long way in helping me feel sexy when naked and during sex. This man of mine is a saint. I've never once felt like a freakshow in front of him.

Okay, that's a lie. The first time they removed the bandages after my mastectomy, I held my breath and looked over at him. His poker face was solidly intact. Since then, he's been a little bit like, "been there, done that. Nothing can shock me." He's also really good at poker. If he were a writer of *how to* books, his might be *How to Treat a Woman and Keep Your Poker Face No Matter What*. I'm a lucky girl. And I can still say *lucky* after the hell I've been through in the name of boobs. The many ways I'm fortunate are not lost on me, I assure you. The first and last thing I do everyday is thank God for the many ways I am truly blessed.

On more than one occasion, plastic surgeons and their staff have responded to my questions about appearance and procedure outcomes with the parental equivalent of "you get what you get, and you don't throw a fit." First of all, who's throwing a fit? And second, your tagline needs some work. I thought a plastic surgeon's job and main endeavor was to make someone look better—their best, even. Wanting to look normal(ish) is no cause for shaming. And it wasn't shaming per se, but I repeatedly heard things like, "you will not look the same," (duh) "we'll see what we can do with what you have to work with," (okay, but what does that even mean?) and "no one is perfectly symmetrical" (I know, but thanks for the newsflash). And who said anything about perfection? That ship sailed with the first mastectomy. And kudos to those plastic surgeons who still have one foot in the elective plastic surgery world as well as the reconstruction world. Maybe because they did plenty of elective cosmetic procedures, I got more understanding from them about my wanting to look good *and* be alive than I did from the ones performing only non-cosmetic, medically necessary procedures.

Sadly, the vibe in the strictly reconstruction world landed much like, "you should be grateful you're alive instead of obsessing about what your chest will look like." Respectfully, fuck off and either get on board or find a new job. Again, this was just a ... vibe I got. None of this was said verbatim. It was more implied, or maybe just how it landed for me. This is where women surgeons may have an edge on men; they get it. And even when the majority of surgeons miss the boat on bedside manner, a fellow woman can at least (hopefully) put herself in your shoes, mostly. There is still this undercurrent of acceptable Frankenstein-ing. I mean, if they are committed to making me look my best, then their elevator pitch might need some fine tuning.

I may sound like a Negative Nelly right now, and I'm not really feeling all the negativity I'm spewing, but there is a significant dark side to all of this that I feel called to shout from the rooftops. I'm convinced if every doctor lived their patient's experience, it would bring a whole new perspective to the table. And it's time to level up already. There has to be a better way. I'm convinced there already is, and I have my guesses on why we're not seeing it. But this isn't that book. There are plenty out there from qualified experts on the subject, so I'll stay in my lane.

With the aforementioned numbers of 150ish medical-related events, it's understandable that some women would opt to just *get what they get and not throw a fit*. Being the squeaky wheel and advocating for yourself is so much more than just the appointments I attended physically and via video. It's waiting on hold for hours to even get the appointments. Yes, hours! It's driving time to and from the appointments—most times, one appointment for me was an all-day event. It's keeping it all straight and keeping life from falling through cracks while you're doing it. And we'll just leave the expense out of it for now. The grind of my body drama is exhausting. On more than one occasion, I've just wanted to stop, throw in the towel and leave it all up to fate. But I don't subscribe to the fate ideology, remember? So I persevered, in the name of boobs.

Looking in the mirror every day and seeing what cancer had taken from me—the reminder of every infusion and radiation appointment, the *event* that was getting dressed every day, trying to find clothes that felt cute but camouflaged the freakshow—motivated me. My driving force? I wanted my body back! A body that could throw on a T-shirt and jeans and fly out the door, wear a swimsuit without constantly thinking about wearing a swimsuit, and most of all, not be reminded of cancer every frickin' minute of every frickin' day. And these are just the surface things.

Under the surface, issues like cording (also known as axillary web syndrome), swelling and tightness in my left arm and the mobility issues it caused, the body aches that made my knees scream even in sleep, stomach issues, the ringing in my ears, and the constant noise in my head are just the highlights of the invisible struggles created by cancer. I don't know about you, but I think it's reasonable to want cancer to take a backseat in life, or maybe ride in the trunk, or fuck it, get out of the car entirely. For me, that desire was enough to keep me going, to see it through to the finish line and hopefully leave it in my rearview mirror for good. Despite missing several once-in-a-lifetime events (including my step dad's funeral) and living like Goldilocks—needing everything *just right* (referencing the ridiculous list of lymphedema risks I must now avoid)—I was determined to realize a new life on the other side of breast cancer and breast reconstruction that resembled the girl I used to know. For me, that was more than reason enough to stay the course.

And there might've been a simpler route, but not for me.

Chapter 4

Implants, Immune System, and Cancer Cells

"Don't take criticism from the cheap seats."
~ Brené Brown

Fortunately for me, my most recent (and God willing, last) plastic surgeon lives in both worlds of *beautiful* plastics and *necessary* plastics. She doesn't currently perform any elective cosmetic surgeries, but does seem to want the best possible outcome when doing necessary reconstruction. She is realistic, but is also a micro surgeon capable of mastering the tiniest detail.

Now the big question: why the quest for live boobs over the much simpler surgery of implants? I've got your answers.

Some women have great success with implants. I've also met some who have had nothing but health issues after getting them. For me, simply put, my left implant got wasted after axillary surgery and radiation.

Technically speaking, it developed contracture and began noticeably swelling and tightening. I was going to need it replaced anyway, if I wanted to have a chest that looked and felt normal. The swelling was happening above the implant, giving me a *third boob* effect above the left one. Aesthetically: super attractive! Beyond aesthetics though was the discomfort and my immune system. When there is a foreign object in your body, the immune system is on high alert, so to speak, creating an inflammatory response. It's like, "Hey, did you see this intruder? It must be stopped." Chronic inflammation is a known link to cancer. When we create these environments for our immune system, it's much like keeping the army focused on this *distraction* so it doesn't see the real enemy coming through the front door, like cancer cells. I wanted my immune system "at ease" so it could and would attack any possible chance of recurrence. It's also worth mentioning I've had a lifelong history of sensitivity to foreign substances, i.e. piercings, tape, adhesives, stitches, tattoos, etc. Some people have no issues with things like this. I had one piercing that hadn't completely healed after a year, so I removed it. But I didn't start realizing my sensitivity issues or even acknowledging them until after the scare of cancer. The narrative of my life growing up was mostly that I was a high-maintenance pain in the ass so I learned to ignore things. I want to hug that girl so much right now.

For those who haven't done the deep dives, implants are generally outpatient surgeries with fantastic outcomes. Two completely symmetrical implants have a no-brainer likelihood of producing a close to perfect-looking chest. And the efficiency of outpatient procedures cannot be overstated. Live tissue is subject to so many variables—it's more of a crapshoot because it settles differently. Some tissue survives and some doesn't, which is expected. So there may be cause for follow up procedures, like fat injections to fill in gaps. In my case, a whole flap died, but that is rare according to medical statistics. In fact, I keep reading about how rare *all* of the shit that went wrong with me is. Just lucky, I guess. I know plenty of doctors who would agree. And I in no way mean to dissuade anyone from live tissue reconstruction. On the contrary, I am still glad I went that route. But at the time (multiple times actually), I would ask myself what the hell I was even doing it all for. It did not feel worth it in those moments—I was literally almost dying for boobs. Who does that? Me, apparently. But I kept my eye on the prize: calm immune system, natural breasts, normal(ish) life.

Chapter 5

Lymphedema and the Waiting Game

Patience is not the ability to wait, but the ability
to keep a good attitude while waiting.
~Unknown

I wonder why we don't know who originally said that
quote. Is it because the ability to *keep* a good attitude
while waiting is a bit of a unicorn? I've yet to find anyone
who possesses this ability. At least, not consistently. I,
for one, had plenty to be impatient about.

I dreaded making medical calls. I always have. It
seemed to require a saintly level of patience. It felt like
a game we (patients and medical professionals) played,
except I (the patient) didn't know the rules. I know I
sound like Negative Nelly again—for the record, I have
seen improvements in this recently, or at least the effort
to improve. And trust me, I implemented all my *positive*
thinking tools any time I had to make a call. This
particular morning, before embarking on the dreaded
calls, I'd just read the above inspiration during my

23

morning routine, hoping to infuse some optimism into my day. You see, after I finished chemo and radiation, lymphedema became my biggest hurdle—my squeakiest wheel on the post-treatment grind to get my life back. Just finding the right lymphedema support was a full-time job, and figuring out where to begin to find support was the job within the job. I became hyper-aware of the discomfort, swelling, and tightness associated with the first signs, not to mention the "third boob" issue above my left implant.

It had been an uphill battle to get the answers and help I sought, outside of paying hundreds of dollars to naturopathic doctors that didn't take insurance. (More accurately, insurance did not provide coverage for visits to "those" doctors. Semantics! Either way, I continued to seek answers within the parameters of western medicine, so insurance would pay for it.) As anyone who has done their time in that arena can attest, it's quite the frustrating hamster wheel. It's maddening to me that insurance companies determine the care we can and cannot receive. And they are *not* doctors!

A little backstory here is I'd developed lymphedema from surgery and radiation. It wasn't a severe case, and maybe that was because I was hypervigilant. During and right after radiation, the radiologist repeatedly cautioned me about developing lymphedema and the signs to look for. The images I conjured of grossly swollen limbs drove my vigilance. After I finished radiation, I began noticing tightness, swelling, and subtle changes in my left chest wall, axilla, and arm. Small things—like not seeing veins on the back of my hand or not being able to put on my wedding ring—were the telltale first signs. Seeking treatment through the teaching hospital where

I received radiation treatment seemed to be my shortest route to relief.

Insurance approved twelve visits to the lymphedema therapist. I guess that's the magic number to cure it. Ironically, my lymphedema didn't get that memo. It didn't magically go away once those twelve visits were completed. I had to go back to the referring radiologist to be assessed, and they determined I needed more treatments. Then I needed to get the referral sent to and then received by the therapist, get contacted by the therapist, and finally get scheduled for more treatments. By the time the powers that be finally decided I could have more treatments, the physical therapy building had closed for some building issues. The physical therapist had no place to set up for patients' treatments, so they couldn't offer them. Did you just sigh heavily after reading this? I sighed heavily just typing it, because we both know that sequence of events didn't happen overnight. Back to square one. You can't make this stuff up.

Meanwhile, I'd heard a podcast where the lymphedema specialist being interviewed gave a website where you could look up specialists in your area. She even provided the specific certifications to look for. I took notes. With this list in hand, I prepared to track one down. The first website I looked up did not take insurance and charged between $200 and $700 depending on what you were looking for. I moved to the next one on the list, took a deep breath, and made the call.

That call went like this:

Me: Hi, I found your physical therapist on a lymphedema directory and am wondering about getting in to see her. I've finished cancer treatment, and the specialist I was seeing can't take patients right now due to a building issue. Does your therapist take new patients and accept insurance?

Receptionist: Well, first you'd need a referral from a doctor. Then she will look it over and decide if she wants to treat you or not.

Did I just hear that right? If. She. Wants. To. Just breathe, Carol.

Me: Okay. Well, before I go through getting the referral, can you tell me if she is LANA (Lymphology Association of North America) certified, or if she is a CLT (certified lymphedema therapist)? And if so, does she have experience with chest and trunk lymphedema, or just arms and hands? Because the name of the practice says hand and arm specifically. I mean, I don't know if you get asked that ques—

Her: (cutting me off) No! Not once have I ever been asked that question. And I've been here *five* years!

Yikes! Okay—that's a firm no, then? Because you sound unsure ... damn! And which question exactly was the hard no? Because I asked, like, five.

Me: Okay, but do you know about the certification? Because while I know you said she must decide if she *wants* to treat me, I also must decide if she has the experience and credentials to treat my issues—ideally before I go through the process of a doctor referral and evaluation.

I swear to the lymphedema gods, I used my nice voice (even if my words were a tad bitchy). I think I deserved points for not screaming into the phone that she's a bag of shit for talking to potential patients like that.

Her: No, I don't have that information. Sorry we couldn't help you. Have a good day.
Me: Wow! That's pretty rude.

I'm not sure if she heard me or if she'd already hung up. One can hope.

I will fully admit I was a bit snarky, but c'mon! If I'm giving Phone Girl the benefit of the doubt, maybe she chose her words carelessly when she said "decide if she *wants* to treat you." But there was also the interruption and the dismissiveness. I'm assuming a person who chose to become a physical therapist didn't do it to pick and choose who to help. It's too bad that her calling card, a.k.a. Phone Girl, didn't get that memo. I mean, arguably her main job is to answer the phone and book patients. I'm taking it on faith that being a rude, dismissive bitch to people isn't in the job description. But it was Monday morning, and stormy outside, and maybe her drive to work sucked, and she spilled her coffee, and someone took her parking spot. Maybe she hadn't had her coffee yet, or Starbucks screwed her order up. Or maybe she's just an asshole and hates her life. Either way, that's a hard pass on using that facility for anything, even if the therapist was qualified and *wanted* to treat me and was the nicest PT in the land of PTs.

The fixer in me wanted to save the next caller from the same fate and appeal to Phone Girl's sense of humanity—assuming she had any—and call her back to rationalize. The meaner fixer in me wanted to tell the PT to get a new phone girl, because hers sucks and is sabotaging her business. I kid you not, my brain works like that—save the world, take on shit that isn't yours, blah, blah, fix it, blah. Exhausting. I'm telling you, this may not be scientific, but I meet more people like me who get cancer than those chill people who innately know how to stay in their lane and shrug off the assholes of life. But I digress. I was the priority here, so I immediately regrouped and locked Codependent Carol back in the closet. I've learned painfully over the years what is and is not mine to fix. That default setting runs deep, so it requires effort ... but not as much as it used to.

I got off that call and immediately hit a wall of guilt. I stopped everything to get still and evaluate—a trick I learned in therapy. Let me be clear: I did not feel guilty for telling her she was rude or for hanging up on her. You see, it's all in the perspective. I was so flabbergasted by her attitude that calling her rude and hanging up was the nicest thing I had in me right then. I concluded that it was her shaming me that did it. She shamed me for asking questions, for wanting—no, *needing*—a specific kind of help. Why was I shamed for seeking the right answers for my personal health? How is that okay in the medical world? How is that okay, period? We are repeatedly told throughout school that there are no dumb questions. Yet in the medical world, my questions were routinely met with rudeness and shaming—when I could get a conversation to happen at all. I kid you not, sometimes the hours on hold would result in me hanging up before I ever even reached someone. But I digress.

This is the information age. We no longer must be blindly led by egomaniacal doctors with God complexes—or their phone people. We have access to a lot of the information we seek. We know more now than ever. We are vastly more aware of what we need and want, especially in medical care. We can table the guilt I took on at her shaming for another day, or another book. I recognized it and, rather quickly, put the onus where it belonged and went on with my day. I count it a win that Phone Girl lived to be rude another day. I still feel sorry for the PT that likely has no idea her phone person sucks. I heard a friend's sermon recently where she talked about confidence and that it's a choice. Inside, we feel one way—we can feel all the things, but we *know* something else. Our confidence isn't in what we feel; it's in what we know. *Confidence is a choice! Lean into what I know! And maybe get counseling for what I feel.* Maybe. That would require more deep dives into what I want in my medical professionals. And at the time, I was in the middle of trying to get help for the lymphedema medical issue. One issue at a time, please.

May I quickly share a few of my favorite scriptures on this very topic? A well-timed scripture can ground me, give me perspective, and get me back on track. Three are among some of my favorites:

"I remain confident of this: I will see the goodness of the Lord in the land of the living." (Psalms 27:13 NIV)

"For I know the plans I have for you, declares the Lord, plans to prosper you and not to harm you, plans to give you hope and a future." (Jeremiah 29:11 NIV)

"Ask and it will be given to you; seek and you will find; knock and the door will be opened to you." (Matthew 7:7 NIV)

My eldest daughter said this to me recently: if God loves us all equally, then He is working in all of us. He has plans for *all* of us. This reminder helps me chill out when I'm met with rude people or want to be rude myself. There is goodness in all of us, even if it doesn't always look like it. If I can keep this mindset in the forefront, I believe it will help me navigate life with more grace.

I continued to find my own solutions to the lymphedema issues while I waited for the PT to get her building back. Granted, my situation wasn't dire. My lymphedema was diagnosed by a professional as Stage 1. I had minimal swelling in my left arm and trunk area surrounding my axilla region. I admit that most people are probably not as vigilant as I am. They probably live their lives unaware of the little things until they become the big things. But frankly, having some limb or area of my body become grossly swollen for life scared the crap out of me, so I noticed everything: the tightness, the immobility, the puffiness, and the heaviness. At times, it felt like I was carrying a folded-up magazine under my arm, or like my arm was too heavy to carry around. An easy, telltale sign of lymphatic swelling is the veins on the back of your hand disappearing, or rings feeling too tight and leaving indents on your fingers. Like I said, little things, slight things the average bear might miss. But I wasn't the average bear. I was a dog with a bone.

I found a helpful CLT on Instagram. She freely shared so much awesome content, and even responded to my direct message asking if she knew of any CLTs in my area. She sent me a list, but all I found were CLTs who did not take insurance and, again, charged anywhere from $200 to $700 per session. I wasn't prepared to pay that amount out of pocket when insurance would cover it—albeit after jumping through their hoops of referral red tape. I continued to follow her posted advice and tried all her techniques on my own until I saw my oncologist for a routine visit. She let me know the physical therapy clinic was back up and running. I began hoop-jumping to get access to new appointments.

It's worth mentioning that the last time I visited their facility, we were deep into the COVID-19 pandemic and things were just weird—totally different than previous appointments. I say this because I'm still not sure what changed. At my new appointment, my original PT spent most of the hour typing on the computer and leaving the room to go get more *stuff*—wraps, tools, etc. She spent maybe a total of ten minutes treating me, and that's a generous estimate. I left there no better off than I showed up. *But insurance and the facility were getting paid, so I guess we're good.*

I left there beyond frustrated and unsure where to turn for help. I drove an hour each way to get to these appointments, so I didn't see the need to keep doing it for ten minutes of treatment. I mentioned the pandemic because I thought maybe she was scared to touch me. Sounds absurd, I know, but hospitals and medical facilities were still over the top with the anti-germ protocol, and this PT came in wearing damn near full hazmat gear. The difference between that appointment and previous ones made no sense. I know that might seem like an assumptive stretch, but we had already witnessed the country collectively lose its freaking mind, so nothing seemed too far fetched at that point. I found out later that she was set to retire, so maybe it was a bit of short-timer syndrome. I guess it doesn't matter what the issue was, except that I was still at my wit's end for finding solid help. She did however, make sure I got referred to a specialist at another teaching hospital in my area that specialized in lymphedema and lymph node transplants, for which I *might be* a candidate. Again, there was a wait involved—especially due to the pandemic.

A month or two later, I received a check-in call from a patient facilitator and got to vent about the CLT situation at their hospital. She got me referred yet again to a new PT they had who was taking over for the retiree. She wasn't lymphedema certified, but was learning lymphedema techniques. With no other options on the horizon and still waiting to get into the specialist, I tried to schedule with her right away. Of course, the therapy order had expired by then and I had to start all over with the hoop-jumping to get the doctor referral, the insurance approval, and finally the appointment. I saw her twice. She was still learning at that first point and, frankly, her energy conveyed that. She talked nonstop and, while very kind and sweet, didn't do much to alleviate my symptoms. I left there both times on the verge of tears and an anxiety attack.

Did I mention that stress can exacerbate swelling in lymphedema patients? One of the items on my Goldilocks list to avoid. I vowed to prioritize simplifying things thenceforth. Then, my stepdad got diagnosed with Stage 4 lung cancer.

Hello, trigger! No stress there!

Of course, there is no genetic link. That wasn't the trigger. The cancer diagnosis itself was undoubtedly part of it, but it was mostly linked to the *cancerism* of unresolved trauma and what some in the cancer world refer to as *issues in the tissues.* My relationships with both my dads are complicated, and I would venture to say that most of my *issues* and trauma stem from them. Although they were both rocky, I had positive, healed relationships with both of them before they died. Facing their deaths, especially my stepdad's, brought up a lot of unresolved trauma, though—even stuff I thought I'd successfully resolved years before. But I'll get back to that a little later.

For the record, I believe in counseling. I've been counseled repeatedly and effectively throughout the years. Don't shoot me here (or stop reading), but my biggest issue with finding a counselor or therapist is the human element. Aren't they all just flawed human beings like us, trying to figure out their own shit? That may sound quite pessimistic, but work with me here.

The cancer medical world does try. It does. I randomly got calls from case workers affiliated with the hospital I got treatment at. They'd check in on me, listen to me rant, and genuinely be supportive. I'd feel better after venting, even though nothing got resolved. They'd provide contacts for anything I felt would help, and counseling was always top of their list of suggestions. There was just so much to wade through post cancer that I regularly felt overwhelmed to the point of paralysis. That's my typical MO when I feel overwhelmed—do nothing and check out. But I didn't do *nothing,* exactly. Remember I mentioned I'd had 150+ appointments in four years of treatment/ two years of reconstruction? Well, I'd had about fifty up to that point. Trust me when I say it was easy to get overwhelmed and simply shut down. I still suffered from chemo brain fog and a plethora of other physical issues that piled on to the already-piled-on pile. Fatigue and lack of motivation were taking the lead. And *one more* doctor's appointment—a regularly repeated one at that—felt like the apple that would tip the cart.

On several occasions, I would go down the rabbit hole of trying to find a counselor or therapist based on the recommendations of the hospital, and a few friends and family members. Committed to my health and good at following medical advice, I'd spend hours reading bios and rejecting all of them for one reason or another. I admit, I was being very picky. The vulnerability it took for this recovering perfectionist/control freak to even seek counseling was greater than what was required for dating in my twenties—way before the internet and social media deep dives existed. Every attempt at finding one was a blind date by today's standards, even when you knew them. My criteria for dating a counselor didn't seem off the charts to me, but was apparently a tall order. I wanted someone with cancer experience, who had Christian beliefs, and who was a woman. And I was open to gray areas—like, maybe she had medical trauma experience, but not necessarily cancer. Or perhaps she didn't claim Christianity, but also didn't ascribe to any specific religious background surrounding her practice. Being a woman was my non-negotiable. I've learned through experience that no one gets the female parts *thing* like a woman. Even incredibly empathetic men give a valiant effort but fall short. Sorry, guys.

"No uterus, no opinion."
~Rachel Green, *Friends*.

For the record, I have no uterus—now. But I used to, so it counts. *Right?*

Finally, I found someone I could see myself talking to week after week. I took a deep breath and booked the appointment. I put it in my calendar and prepared myself for the grind and deep digging of therapy. This may not be the normal response to impending therapy, but I am nothing if not thorough. If I'm going to get in there and figure shit out, I'm going all in. I'd always viewed therapy as a daunting but worthwhile task. A couple hours before my appointment, I got a message that the *chosen one* wouldn't be available and had to cancel my appointment. Look, I'm not a complete asshole. I believe there was some life stuff that happened over there, and it was unavoidable. But we hadn't even had our first date yet. I just couldn't, in good conscience, start our relationship on a flaky note. And that was the nail in the coffin for me on therapy—for this cancer journey, anyway. Besides, I had some solid support in my life, and they didn't charge me or need a referral. Maybe a meal or a few drinks and a bit of my standup routine on coping with difficult shit through deflective and self-deprecating humor was all I needed. Either way, I was done with the blind dates. And frankly, it was a relief to take one spoke of doctors' visits off the hamster wheel.

I was also still in that holding pattern, trying to get into the specialist/surgeon at that other teaching hospital. That surgeon's office had finally called to get me in, but with the COVID-19 pandemic, he was only doing video appointments. I declined at first, asking them to let me know when he resumed in-person appointments, which cost me months of delay. I thought it would be pointless to see him on video. How could he truly assess my lymphedema through a computer screen? I learned from a friend in the industry that I needed to take that appointment to officially become his patient. Then, he *had* to help me. "That's the game," she revealed. Who knew? I do now. And so do you.

When I did eventually get to see him on video, he proved to be a wealth of knowledge and options. The biggest option was a lymph node transplant, which would allow my left side to function more normally and hopefully without the daily use of wraps, bandages, and compression. Sign me up! I didn't even know all of what it entailed, but I knew I wanted in. I had a severe intolerance to compression garments and was allergic to most adhesive. The compression caused more swelling, instead of reversing or stopping it. It took my high sensitivity to a whole new level. This was not even the tip of the iceberg, I assure you—unbeknownst to me. I clung to the hope of making my body function normally again. He approved me as a candidate for a lymph node transplant, an explant surgery (the removal of implants), and live tissue flap reconstruction with the plastic microsurgeon on his team. Cue the next waiting game to see the next rockstar on the team.

As I said, the whole reason I needed lymphedema therapy was because radiation and surgery on my axilla (armpit) caused swelling, tightness, immobility in my shoulder area, and contracture to my implant. However, not one time did the doctor-appointed, insurance-approved therapist address or touch my contracture or chest/trunk area. They paid all their attention to my arm and hand, and they were constantly coming up with new compression garments—expensive garments to buy and try. Gloves, sleeves, wraps, and bandages—all of which were not returnable once you bought them. So, the whole *try and buy* thing was really just *buy and good luck*. One thing they did suggest for my trunk was a tight-fitting camisole that I'd need to wear 24/7. So naturally, I'd need two so I could wear one while the other was being washed—*every day*.

As I mentioned earlier, compression didn't work on me like it was supposed to. My fingers would swell up three times their size and turn purple, which they told me meant I needed a different garment or a different size. More purchases of nonreturnable items. I took this horseshit for a few months. I'd already stopped being able to wear my wedding ring and my Apple watch. I'd even resized my wedding ring in hopes of being able to wear it. The watch later became a hand-me-down to my daughter, a new college athlete who could put it to good use. The jeweler and I decided to make the ring slightly bigger than I needed in case I had more swelling. That necessitated the use of rubber sizers. If I didn't use the exact amount of rubber coils, the ring was either too loose or too tight. I mostly didn't wear it, as I didn't want to lose it or risk more swelling.

For special occasions, I would suck it up and wear it and usually end up looking for a safe place to stash it in my purse when I had to take it off halfway through the event. I did say shitshow, didn't I? The wearing of my wedding ring became a whole *thing*. The ring situation was bordering on stress—or, at the very least, an overthinking issue. It began staying in the jewelry box, even on special occasions. And I love my wedding ring! But lymphedema swelling can be permanent if not caught early and treated. It didn't seem worth the risk. The whole thing pissed me off. It was just one more thing. I wanted my body to act normally. I also wanted to wear my ring. I don't wear a lot of jewelry, anyway—my ring and some diamond studs from my husband. That's it. And it may sound overdramatic, but I felt naked without them. Cancer had taken enough already. Can I just wear my damn ring? And can I get some actual help for the lymphedema? It's incredible to me how much we don't know about lymphedema, considering how prevalent breast cancer is and how often the treatment for said breast cancer causes it.

In between my physical therapy treatments, I also experimented with other forms of therapy, including an expensive compression pump. It seemed to work for a minute, until it didn't. Then it began exacerbating the swelling. That new development (and an unfortunate visit to the compression garment store) became the first nail in the coffin for insurance-approved lymphedema support. The store owner would not accept that my body didn't respond to compression like all her training told her it should. She shamed me that I wasn't doing my due diligence. I wore the latest suggested garment (a glove and arm sleeve), along with the everpresent camisole, to what became my last appointment. It was an hour drive for me. As I drove, I watched my fingers swell and swell. I took pictures to document it. Once they began to change colors—first red, then purple—I took a quick picture and, completely freaked out by the visual, removed all the compression. This was done in stop-and-go commuter traffic safely, when I was stopped.

By the time I arrived for my appointment, my fingers had almost returned to normal. One of the store owner's employees, an extremely compassionate and sweet woman I liked from our first meeting, sympathized with me and wanted to refund me for the garments and try to find another solution. She was looking up Facebook groups I could join and doing her best to get me answers while we waited for the owner. She needed the owner to come in and assess me to see if she could offer something more—a.k.a. approve a refund. That's when the shaming started. The owner came in like a force—authoritative, and like a teacher talking to an ignorant student. She wanted me to put the garments back on and sit there for an hour so she could see for herself. I showed her the pictures to *prove* I wasn't lying. She stood her ground on wanting to see it for herself, and began suggesting new, alternative garments. At that point, I'd had enough. My side of the conversation went something like this:

"I've shown you pictures. I don't think I should have to be your human guinea pig and risk permanent swelling, wasting an additional hour of my time and yours, just so you can verify what I've already shown you. And now you're suggesting more expensive garments when the hundreds of dollars in non-returnable garments I've already purchased aren't working. I realize it's frustrating that I'm a rare person compression is not working for like you'd expect—"

Cutting me off and turning to her employee, she said, "Just return them and give her the money back."

Then, not bothering to look at me once, she turned and left the room, closing the door behind her. All I can say is it's a good thing she left. I was furious! I seriously don't understand people who choose to work in healthcare but aren't more empathetic. As I type this, I envision putting a schoolyard smackdown on this chick. But pounding on someone, I'm quite sure, isn't good for lymphedema. Otherwise ...

The nice employee and I looked at each other like deer in headlights. She then began talking and trying to do whatever it is you're supposed to do when your boss is an asshole, and you are not. I began reeling in my shock and trying to listen to her words. She took the garments back and gave me a full refund. As she was processing all of that, she dropped some nuggets of gold on me. I'd curiously asked when I'd be in the clear of developing lymphedema. She told me it is a lifetime ordeal that can develop at any time, and described two cases where the patients had developed lymphedema at ten and fifteen years post surgery and treatment. When I asked what they'd done differently or how it happened, she said one got a vaccine and the other got a tattoo. She further explained that doing *anything* that could create an immune response in your body can trigger it. I was back to the deer in the headlights as my mind reeled with scenarios.

By the way, the checklist for lymphedema dos and don'ts is quite extensive. Think the Princess and the Pea on steroids. They gave me a handout with a bulleted list of over thirty items to avoid:

- lifting heavy objects
- restrictive garments like bra straps
- jewelry like watches and rings
- blunt force
- extreme temperatures
- pedicures/manicures
- hot tubs/saunas/steam rooms above 105 degrees
- cuts
- insect bites
- altitude changes
- gardening
- tennis

Just to name a few.

Oh, and they suggest elevating the afflicted arm when traveling and sleeping. *Hmmm ...*

For an overthinker like me, the noise in my head was deafening:

Can I still wear my wedding ring? Can I carry my own groceries? If I cut my finger slicing limes, should I be worried? I mean, I am, but ... How in the hell do I avoid insect bites? I mean, that's always the goal, isn't it? But I'm guessing the insect world doesn't get the memo of who's off limits. No traveling to the tropics? The snow? Sweating at a ballgame, or the gym? Pedicures?

Seriously? How do I sleep with my arm elevated, anyway? And let's forget about the lymphedema for a second—did I eat more good food than bad today? Did I exercise enough? I didn't do the yoga breathing. All this stressing isn't helping me. Just breathe, Carol! They got it all. You did all the treatments. You're cancer-free. You're healed. You're healthy. You're well, in Jesus' name. Please, God, light the path to health and healing. Lead me to good doctors. To answers. To the right answers. But how will I know what the right answers are? Ugh—God, what's your stance on lobotomies?

I began my own search for lymphedema support outside of traditional medicine. I grudgingly resolved to continue seeing the new therapist who was still learning, in hopes something was better than nothing. It turns out that between her canceling on me and me canceling on her for various reasons, I never did see her again. This was when I found that Certified Lymphedema Therapist online who generously shared her wisdom and knowledge on Instagram. Her handle is *thepinkpros* if you're interested. As I mentioned, I did all the exercises she demonstrated and researched the list of nearby providers she shared with me. It's important to know that I live in a rural town and every appointment would be a minimum of an hour's drive away. My experiences with the list were unsuccessful, not covered by insurance, incredibly expensive, and—in that one experience—exceptionally rude.

I've since discovered that the standard rate is closer to $100/hour—not completely unreasonable. And while they don't take insurance, you can try to get your insurance to reimburse you. I've not had luck with that so far and frankly, have mostly given up trying. I'm picking my battles and dialing down the stress, I guess. Already overwhelmed with the sheer amount of legwork involved in my own care, my stress levels were high—and subsequently, so was the swelling. I relied heavily on exercises I found online and doing whatever I could to keep my life as stress-free as possible. Breathwork, prayer, journaling, gratefulness, and mindfulness were huge components of my daily routine while I waited for the referral appointment to see the plastic surgeon. As I said, I didn't know what a lymph node transplant entailed, but I loved the idea of having a working lymph system to repair what radiation and surgery had compromised. I underestimated the wait time to see a rockstar. Life conveniently provided plenty of distractions during my wait.

A trip to celebrate my eldest daughter graduating from college was easily the nicest one. We had a week of celebrations and activities planned a state away from my reminders of cancer, treatments, and all those appointments. The things I couldn't escape, I dragged around with me. As I've repeatedly said, stress can exacerbate it. So, worrying about swelling and triggers for swelling can, in themselves, cause swelling. There's a catch-22 cliché in there somewhere. There was also the everpresent plethora of side effects from the aromatase inhibitor, a hormone blocker I'd been prescribed to take for five to ten years following treatment. Some people have zero side effects. As a highly sensitive person, I had no such luck. I had debilitating joint aches, crippling "trigger finger" on both hands, severe fatigue, anxiety, and depression. I'm probably leaving some out, but those were the stars of the show. I was so excited to see our kids and celebrate our graduate, and I just wanted to feel good during the trip.

During our visit with them a few months before that, I had a moment. I later found out it was a suicidal ideation moment. I'd heard the term before, but never put any thought into what it meant. It's one of those things you may hear spoken out loud, but because it's not a factor for you personally, it doesn't resonate. Turns out it wasn't even my first time having one of those moments, but back then I must've chalked it up to severe teenage angst and/or hormones. Funnily, hormones (or lack thereof) were a factor this time around, too. It's worth mentioning that I have worked hard on knowing and recognizing my triggers, to keep my life on as even a keel as possible—especially while on these wicked anti-cancer drugs that, according to oncologists, were non-negotiable. It's worth mentioning that some integrative, naturopathic, and holistic practitioners refer to these drugs as low-dose chemo. Western medicine doctors do not. I can attest that the side effects make them at least a first cousin.

On that visit, our kids had just picked us up from the airport and we stopped off at our favorite ice cream shop on the hour-long drive back to their house. Ice cream is one of those things I avoided as much as possible, post cancer—it was part of my "cancer/peace of mind" protocol. And I love ice cream. It should be a major food group, right alongside pizza and Mexican food. On the drive there, I was examining my hand for flight-induced swelling and doing a manual lymphatic drainage massage in my seat. I was telling myself that enjoying ice cream with the family is a joyous occasion and *would not* give me cancer. When we arrived at the ice cream shop, it was busy and loud. Thanks to chemo-induced tinnitus, my hearing wasn't what it used to be, especially in loud places. I missed some inside joke the kids and my husband made, and they were all laughing.

When I asked what I missed, they blew me off and said it was nothing. I internally flipped my shit. Everything went tunnel vision and buzzy. I excused myself to go to the bathroom while they waited in line. I used the bathroom while I tried to get my wits about me. While washing my hands and looking in the mirror, a voice in my head said they'd be better off without me. No more accommodating hoops to jump through for the high-maintenance pain in the ass I'd become.

My oldest daughter is highly sensitive and zeros in on the emotional current in the room. When I opened the bathroom door, she was standing there, waiting. She said, "I'm going to use it too, come in with me." I'm sure she could tell I was trying not to cry and started to talk in the way she does when she wants to make something better or distract someone. I let her, because I wanted to feel better, and I wanted my family to enjoy themselves. I remember the strange experience of seeing my mom cry as a kid—even an adult kid. As a mom, I always want to protect my kids. As a mom with a shit-ton of issues, I also want to spare them my "legacy." And most importantly, I knew my doom thoughts were fake. I knew it, despite being unable to stop them. I'd had enough experience with depression, anxiety, and therapy to know this was not me but the drugs.

A few months later, when it was time for our next trip—the graduation trip—I knew I wanted to feel good, be present, and enjoy all the festivities. My oncologist from the hospital where I did my infusions mentioned once that people take hormone blocker "holidays" when they have something important to do. I was now under the care of a new oncologist at the closer hospital that I'd had radiation at. I asked her about the holiday thing. She was not a fan. She did not greenlight the break. I decided to give myself the break anyway because I knew of one oncologist who did support it—and she wasn't just any oncologist. She was a highly sought after leading breast cancer specialist at a nationally ranked, top ten hospital. Based on what she'd said, I felt comfortable doing it without my current oncologist's approval. And I'm not one to break the rules willy nilly. If she hadn't been an additional hour or two away from me than my current oncologist, she'd still be my oncologist. All that to say, I trusted her opinions and protocol.

The difference I felt on that trip compared to how I'd been progressively feeling over the last two years was night and day. I felt like myself again. My pain was minimal and my mood was calmer and happier— genuinely happier. I found myself again. I couldn't go back. I didn't race right out and tell the new oncologist; I waited until my next appointment to break the news. I didn't ask permission; I told her it was happening. She went from essentially forbidding it, to accepting and semi-supporting my decision. And believe me, I weighed my decision, but it didn't take long at all for me to make it. I concluded that I'd rather risk not taking the drug and be happy and present and ... me, than be depressed, in pain, and feeling like my world would be better off without me. Easy decision to my way of thinking. But again, I'm not usually a rule breaker. I tightened up my diet and absolutely felt justified removing certain things from my life in the name of health and peace, and became more relaxed about everything.

For the record, I do not suggest trying to change a diet in one fell swoop. I highly recommend a moderate, slow, and steady approach. It has a much better success rate of becoming a lifestyle. And I do support and strongly suggest everyone getting on board the healthy lifestyle train. I don't see how people do not connect the dots between their diets and their health.

A few of my hard-and-fast diet changes included:

- Knowing where the meat comes from (if you eat meat). Hormone-free, grass-fed and finished, cage-free, free-range, humanely raised, and antibiotic-free are some of the non-negotiable things I look for. If I don't know where it's from, I mostly don't eat it.
- Following a mostly whole foods diet, which means no highly processed food. Highly processed food isn't food anyway. What plant is a Cheeto from? By the way, cheese is a highly processed food. Don't shoot the messenger. I love cheese. I just don't eat it very much anymore.
- Reading labels. More than ten ingredients is too many. I have to know what the ingredients are and be able to pronounce them.
- Knowing what inflammatory foods are and staying away from them, like bad oils (corn, canola, and seed oils). Good oils are olive, avocado, and coconut.

- Knowing what anti-inflammatory foods are and eating them as much as possible.
- Limiting sugar in all its forms (except for berries), especially processed sugar.
- Following an 80/20 rule. Eighty percent of the time doing it right. Twenty percent of the time, letting myself indulge. Stressing about it might be worse than indulging.
- When out in the world, not overthinking it. If the restaurant isn't the healthiest, I try to order a salad—or hit the "fuck it" button and get fries. But I eat home-cooked meals, mostly.
- Limiting alcohol and caffeine.
- Remembering that nothing tastes as good as cancer-free feels. Read that again!

The average person may say "why couldn't she have done that to begin with?" And that, my friends, is the million-dollar question. If we could all do that, I believe with every fiber of my being that there would be less illness, disease, and premature death in this world. But is there even really an average, issue-less person? I think not. In this era of highlight reels, fear of missing out (FOMO), and new levels of keeping up with the Joneses—and *knowing* the Joneses and every piece of their business—don't we all have issues? Frankly, it seems we may have issues more than we have anything else. But I digress.

When I finally got in to see the plastic microsurgeon, I'd waited almost a year. At that initial appointment, I wasn't even going to get to meet her, at first. I met her nurse and proverbial right hand. She came in full of energy and passion for her job—a plus. But she matter-of-factly explained how they'd remove my belly fat and skin, along with my navel and my favorite tattoo, stretch and pull down the skin, make a new navel, and use all the belly fat they removed to make boobs. "Horrified" is an understatement. Even my husband's poker face faltered for a second after she casually threw out how the tattoo on my hip (my wedding flower) would "mostly" be gone— "Well, at least half of it." *Wait, what?!*

"So, you're going to possibly leave half a tattoo on my body?" I asked incredulously.

Aren't we trying to dial down the freak show?

Breezing over that, she said my stomach will look flat, like that would sufficiently resolve the issue. What part of leaving a frankensteined tattoo on my body did she not get? I wanted her to say something to put me at ease. After repeatedly trying to sell me on it, she brought in the big guns, but even the plastic surgeon couldn't sway me. It all sounded barbaric. I left there asking for more options, asking what else the surgeon could do. She threw out some hasty alternative plans, but I felt like I was on a car lot. I wasn't interested in the top-of-the-line model so they weren't as interested in selling me the cheaper version. I'm not saying that was the case, it's just how it was landing for me at the time. I want to believe that was not the case. I'm choosing to believe that.

After months of waiting, I finally got my answers: I would not have enough excess fat taken from liposuction alone to create anything beyond a flat chest. I nervously agreed to the original plan and cost myself months by not agreeing to it right away. This is where that elevator pitch comes in handy. Sell it better! Maybe don't scare the shit out of the new potential patients because you are so used to talking about and executing this barbaric shit on a daily basis like it's *no big deal*. Just food for thought. And it's worth mentioning that this nurse was the kindest, most caring nurse I'd ever worked with. Truly compassionate. Again, I think it's like going nose blind to certain smells in our own homes. They do this every day. They forget how horrific it all sounds to the mere mortals. I in no way mean to bash her. She has been my biggest advocate in all of this by far. But also, maybe with all this creative plastic surgery, we can also figure out how to remove an *entire* tattoo and not delve into abstract art while we're at it. I made sure to clarify that at my next visit, and the tattoo was removed entirely. It's a bummer it had to be removed at all, because it was by far my favorite. I would have gladly traded all my others to take its place.

This microsurgeon was a rockstar but a bit of a mixed bag for me. I was in awe of what she did and can do. I loved that she did incredible medical things for less fortunate women in other countries. She was articulate, cute, and sometimes funny. But I was beyond frustrated in her lack of planning, orchestrating, and executing of the reconstruction projects under her watch. I've since learned a bit about the moving parts involved in pulling off these procedures, including booking ORs, scheduling pre-ops with surgeons and anesthesiologists, and scheduling post-op appointments. The post-ops were with PAs (physician's assistants) or NPs (nurse practitioners) instead of the rockstar, because the rockstar was almost always operating on someone else. There was also the juggling required, as she traveled to other countries for months at a time to perform surgeries for less privileged people than me. Which brings me back to the feelings of guilt and entitlement that go along with wanting to have a successful outcome and timely resolution to this massive machine that is breast reconstruction. The stops and starts of my own ordeal were mind-blowing, and I'm just one of many. I've overheard similar frustrations in waiting rooms, so I'm definitely not the only one. This seems to be the *modus operandi.*

Even if you have the picture-perfect experience with none of the detour routes I had to take, this is still a years-long commitment. It is not for the faint of heart, I assure you. And before you go all-in on that outpatient implant route, know that breast implant illness is a real thing, though it is largely unrecognized and difficult to diagnose. They usually diagnose it by ruling out everything else. And I'm just going to say it, it can accompany a lot of gaslighting and feeling like you're going crazy to get there. I do not have personal experience with this, but I have friends and acquaintances I've talked to in depth who have. Once the implants were removed, their symptoms and issues largely resolved. It didn't happen overnight, but it did happen. Not to belabor the immune system piece, but the inflammation created by the foreign objects in our bodies keep the immune system on high alert over something we've put there, not a true enemy exactly. But it distracts the immune system from doing what it's designed to do: eliminate or neutralize the bad stuff. Speaking of bad stuff ...

Chapter 6

Epigenetics and the Issues in My Tissues

Trauma is not what happens to you, it's what happens inside you as a result of what happens to you.
~Dr. Gabor Maté

Pause with me while I jump back to the issues in my tissues.

You know that saying, "better the devil you know?" Well, time has a way of wearing you down and making you forget what the truth of a situation really was. Like a fish story in reverse—it doesn't get bigger with time, it somehow diminishes. Kind of like childbirth—if we didn't get over the intense pain and recover, there'd be no siblings. I've learned (and experienced firsthand) that victims of trauma and abuse can sometimes gaslight themselves into remembering it as being less traumatic than it was. A form of survival, maybe ...

Anyone in the cancer world has likely heard the term "the issues are in the tissues." This means that unresolved trauma will stay with us and manifest in other ways—mainly illness and disease. They even have a name for it: epigenetics, the study of how our behaviors and environment can cause changes that affect the way our genes work. Unlike genetic changes, epigenetic changes are reversible and do not change your DNA sequence, but they can change how your body reads a DNA sequence. Which is a fancy way of saying ... we got issues.

Let me be transparent here: I don't just have issues, I have subscriptions of issues. Granted, I've worked through many of them throughout my adult life, especially after being diagnosed with cancer. I did, and do, many things to feel like I'm controlling what I can control to prevent recurrence. But digging through my bag of dysfunctional crap feels much like trying to clean up a hoarder's house. You open one drawer, and it leads to more drawers.

My biggest drawer that houses all the other drawers is probably my membership in Generation X. The comedy bit of my generation is that we were all raised on hose water and neglect. While funny, I can confirm the accuracy. No disrespect to our parents. They (mine, anyway) just worked a lot—they had to—so we were left mostly to our own devices. And if we didn't happen to work our shit out before parenthood (or maybe even if we did), we became a generation of helicopter parents, trying to be the parents we needed when we were young.

I could entertain you with all my GenX crazy, but that would be a whole other book. I'll just give you the highlight reel, which goes something like this: child of divorce with daddy issues stemming from his departure when I was four, a *mean* stepfather I resented, looking for love in all the wrong places (like the country song) from puberty, leading to toxic love relationships into my early twenties—and toxic relationships in general as I worked to be perfect enough to earn the love I sought with friends, siblings, parents, etc. well into my thirties and forties.

The thing about my generation being left to their own devices so often is that most of us never learned how to develop boundaries or form functional relationships. Unlike Millennials, who came after us and have been dubbed as setting too many boundaries. The Baby Boomers who came before us may have set the tone for the overachieving, workaholic, absentee parenting we experienced. Maybe we were the original latchkey kids, because Boomers didn't lock their doors yet. Maybe Mayberry was on its way out but hadn't completely disappeared. I mean, we could dig through those drawers ad nauseam. But again, probably a whole other book. So back to my issues ...

Everything this GenXer learned came from the television shows I watched; which romanticized chaos, drama, and happily ever after. Or, worse, I learned from other, equally ill-equipped peers, or by watching my workaholic, dysfunctional parents largely ignore us in their quest to make ends meet. Some of my best memories are of being dropped off at my maternal grandparents' house for weeks on end, where Mayberry was still alive and well, while my mom hustled to bring home the bacon as a struggling single parent—before the evil stepfather entered the picture and after the deadbeat dad bailed.

The "evil" part of "evil stepfather" is simply a nod to my dramatic, *raised-on-MTV* roots. He wasn't exactly evil—at least not all the time. The "deadbeat" part of "deadbeat dad," however, is accurate. *Real dad* never helped support us, monetarily or otherwise. And that is not a dramatic retelling. He literally never paid child support or helped my mom in any way. He'd admit that, too, if he were still alive. In his defense, he had his own issues, namely addiction and alcoholism. I came to realize in my late thirties that the blessing *was* his absence, in that he didn't model that addiction for his kids, up close and personal. The first of only two summers my sister and I ever spent with him included the first of six stepmothers and her twisted kids—it had detrimental and lasting effects on us.

One of the few times my dad visited us, we had to visit in his vehicle in front of our house because this wasn't a television show of the 70s. None of the adults got along, so there were no polite kitchen table conversations over tea and cookies. That stepmother was the woman my dad left us for, so she was jealous of my mom and my mom, justifiably, probably couldn't stand her. This is nothing I can concretely confirm, just the vibe I get from the snippets of memories.

Parked on the curb in front of our house, we let it slip that our stepdad—at the time, her boyfriend—spanked us, and my dad went ballistic, banged on the front door, screamed in my mom's face that he'd kill her and her boyfriend if she ever let him touch his kids again. I remember the stepmother calling after him not to go inside the house as he rushed to the door. I don't remember much else about that visit except a lot of yelling, crying, slamming doors, and drama—and the floating heart necklace my dad gave me that I wore faithfully until it broke sometime in my twenties. In hindsight, both the scene and the necklace seemed to prove to me that despite his inability to stay sober and be present and supportive, he did care about us.

It must have come off that way to my mom too, because shortly after, she let me and my sister stay a whole summer with him and the stepmother and her kids. The only other visits with him were occasional trips to his mom's house, my Nonnie, for long weekends here and there. This stepmother had four of her own kids— two adult girls already on their own, and two teenagers, one boy and one girl, who lived with them. A couple life-changing events happened that summer—which may be the understatement of the year. I'm not even sure how to get into it—there is so much to unpack. And I've never really unpacked it for the masses before. *Lucky you (and me).*

Let me start with this: I was born a thumb sucker. It was my main source of soothing and comfort, even as old as eight or nine—especially since the teddy bear I loved had been sewn back together so many times he was finally *retired* (thrown away) and replaced with a nicer, newer bear that never measured up. That summer, the stepmother decided she was putting a stop to the thumb sucking. She recruited my dad and her two kids into her militant crusade. Everyone was constantly on my ass about it, except my sister, who I didn't know at the time had her own issues. Every time I turned around, all I heard was "don't suck your thumb." Every morning, I would hear the step kids coming up the stairs after waking (I was always the first one up and would be watching cartoons way before any of the other kids stirred, after the grown-ups were already gone to work). I'd suck my thumb until the last possible moment when I knew they'd be turning the corner at the top of the stairs. I'd pull my thumb out of my mouth just in time. Without even looking at me, whichever kid it was, usually the boy, would turn and say, "don't suck your thumb." Even at eight years old, I took immense satisfaction in hearing them stop mid-sentence because they realized I wasn't, in fact, sucking my thumb. So, it was mostly just, "don't suck your ... "

One night, they were babysitting us while my dad and stepmother went out. On their way out the door, the stepmother said, "don't let her suck her thumb. If she does, put socks on her hands." She laid a pair of socks on the TV console as a warning. I'm guessing these two teenagers couldn't wait to be in charge. They waited to catch me sucking my thumb. It was close to bedtime, and I guess I was too tired to remember to play the game of beating them to the punch. As soon as I was caught, they ordered me to wear the socks. I refused. They tried to then forcibly put them on me. As soon as they succeeded, I defiantly took them off. *They weren't the boss of me.* They chased me down the stairs to the bedroom my sister and I shared, tackled me on the bed, held me down, and forced the socks onto my hands again. I screamed and cried and thrashed and fought. In my young mind, she was a monster and so were her kids. But they scared me enough that I left the socks on my hands, even after they left me alone, crying, on the bed.

The triggers of this event have lasted all my life and frankly, are breaking me down as I type this. There are so many levels of wrong here, layers and layers. The most obvious basic one being that my one source of comfort was stripped away from me, violently, in a place that wasn't my home and without my mom. The more nuanced issues were shaming a kid for *having* the comforting habit in the first place, and attacking (literally) then punishing said kid for using it. Kids lack the life experience to reason through shit like this. In my innocence, I was subconsciously learning that soothing and comforting myself was not okay. I was learning that feeling comforted and soothed was not okay. I was learning not to trust the adults in my life to keep me safe. I couldn't articulate any of this, but it left its indelible mark. I began chewing my nails off until they bled. I subconsciously welcomed the pain, though it would sometimes make it hard to use my fingers to do things. I've often wondered about the psychology of it, possibly being that the physical pain helps numb the emotional pain of whatever the issue is: trauma, abuse, low self-esteem, family conflict, and/or bullying. I don't know and haven't done the deep dives on it or discussed it in depth in therapy, but when I see a kid chewing off their nails, it gives me a moment of pause, a wave of sadness, and even a slight tightening in my chest.

I wish I could tell you that was the height of the summer trauma. It was just the beginning. My mom had studied cosmetology and loved to keep our hair long to do fun braids and ponytails with. My stepmonster cut our hair off that summer without permission into what they called the Dorothy Hamill, more commonly known as the wedge cut. This meant our just-above-our-butts-length hair was cut to just below our ears. It was super trendy and probably adorable. But I thought I looked like a boy. They (so we) also moved that summer from

Monterey, California to Los Angeles, California. My mom agreed to let us stay with them approximately three hours away and then he moved to a place that was over seven hours away. That would prove to be an issue when it came time to get us back. And—not to bury the lead, but unbeknownst to me, the stepbrother had been *behaving inappropriately* toward my sister. I can't really say much more about that because it isn't my story to tell, and she didn't tell anyone until we were in our thirties. The final traumatic thing that happened is that my mom was forced to come get us at the end of the summer in the middle of the night, with police assistance. "If you want them back, you're going to have to come and get them."

For weeks before the *pickup*, my dad would ask us who we wanted to live with. We, of course, would say him. Kids want to please their parents. He would make us get on the phone and tell our mom that, too. I found out as an adult that, during one such call, my sister waited for my dad and the stepmother to turn their backs long enough for her to whisper into the phone, "come get us."

My mom had been repeatedly asking my dad when he was bringing us back because "school was starting soon." The original agreed-upon arrangement was that he would bring us back at the end of the summer. With her work schedule and being the sole source of income, it was nearly impossible for her to come get us. After that phone call and my sister's plea, she did though, with a police escort who happened to be a family friend and worked for our local police department. We were awakened to hysterical crying, courtesy of the teenage daughter who was inconsolable that we were leaving, though I couldn't figure out why. She didn't even like us. *Drama!*

There were many more minor incidents that pop into my mind even now, but again, I'm just giving the highlights here. In my adult brain, I'm looking back and seeing a shitshow of addiction-led chaos. We came home from that summer changed. My sister developed an eating disorder and a desire to change schools to a place where no one knew her. I came home angry and moody with a slant toward self-hatred when I couldn't pull off the perfectionist tendencies I'd developed. And my mom was a deer in headlights trying to understand what the hell happened to her daughters. Our new attitudes only served to bring out the worst in her boyfriend—not yet the stepfather.

I must mention that my dad spent the last thirty years of his life sober, giving back to the community that helped him get there and reconciling his relationships with his children and my mom. It's worth saying again and again (to others and myself) that we are not the sum of our mistakes and regrets. My heart has nothing but love, forgiveness, and grace for my dad. I feel true peace when I think of him. My stepfather ... that's a heavy, mixed bag.

Guilt is a heavy bag, too and I know my mom carries some for the choices she made. Like letting us spend that first summer with my dad and for staying with my stepdad even after she realized he could be an abusive asshole. Having been in my own blackhole of shitty relationships, I have grace for the blinders she wore and the rose-colored rationale. The thing about abuse is that it can be sneaky—especially if it doesn't come in the form of bruises and black eyes (which for her, it technically did—twice that I know of). As a little kid, he just came off as scary to me and my sister. He worked in law enforcement, so I guess that kind of went with the stereotypical territory. Not cop bashing here. On the contrary, I have a lifelong respect for the sacrifices law enforcement officers make in the name of our safety. But I've met less than I can count on one hand who don't possess that stereotypical, hardass facade. My stepdad, who fit the stereotype to the nth degree, was my main and sometimes only father figure since I was six or seven—for better or worse. And frankly, he was a little bit of both. A silver lining of him being a permanent fixture were the occasional visits with his kids, also two girls. His youngest was exactly my older sister's age, three years ahead of me. And in my young mind, I remember her being the prettiest girl I'd ever seen, and I wanted to be just like her. She also seemed to like me more than my *real* sister did.

Comparing stories on our first camping trip together, we realized a couple things: 1) he was an asshole to them too, smacking them around and being generally scary, and 2) my mom was *the other woman*. And those kids didn't really like us, or her (especially her) as much as I'd thought or hoped. Maybe Cinderella isn't a fairytale. Switch up a few details and we're there: evil stepfather, check! Two evil stepsisters, check, check! Okay, I'm being GenX dramatic here. None of them were evil. But here's the thing about trauma: the people who've been traumatized by someone or something in their past get to decide what is and is not traumatic for them; the people at the root of the trauma do not. And just so we're all on the same page (no pun intended), trauma is not what's happening outside the body, i.e.

circumstances and situations, but what's happening inside us because of what's happening to us or around us. And these responses get hardwired into our nervous systems. It becomes a default operating system, a pattern, a trauma response. An issue!

The first time my stepdad scared the shit out of me was when he "spanked" me and my sister with a rolled-up rope for being ill-mannered, spoiled children and not listening *the first time*. We were spoiled, but that was likely a side effect of a single mom trying to make up for the lack of a dad. We were short on discipline and long on whining to get our way. A solid coping skill among kids from broken homes–not a clinical diagnosis, just an observation. That day, we were playing jump rope in the house—and rather creatively, in my opinion. Since it was just the two of us, we'd tied one end to the doorknob and took turns jumping and *turning*. After being told twice by our mom to stop jumping, he swooped in to come to her defense, took the rope from my sister, who was *turning*, untied it from the door, coiled it up, and whipped us with it. This event cemented my eggshell/rabid dog mentality around him. Walk softly and give it a wide berth. My sister said that's the day she decided she didn't like him, and in almost thirty-nine years of their marriage, she never deviated from that. But that incident leads me to another core memory.

The second *major* time (there were plenty of minors) my stepfather scared the shit out of me was when he hit my mom. I didn't see him do it, just the aftermath. Apparently, a swiftly placed backhand can make the side of someone's face explode. Her black eye, cut lip, and swollen cheek looked like she'd taken a serious beating, but she was quick to tell us he *just* backhanded her. As I was a teenager by then, and more programmed than ever by my television show *therapy*, I couldn't stand that she was downplaying this. As soon as she left the house that day and we were home alone with him, I dramatically climbed out my bedroom window and ran away from home. I could've probably just snuck out the front door. It was a short-lived long weekend of hiding out at my boyfriend's house before I was *dragged* back home under threat of police intervention, thanks to *our* family cop friend—the same cop friend who helped my mom get us back from my dad that long-ago summer. You'd think him having some background would've made him more sympathetic. Not so much. Well, maybe he was, but only toward the adults. I was just an entitled asshole kid who should be more grateful for *the roof over my head.*

Back at home from my *long weekend*, I became more angry, disrespectful and hell bent on defiance. Equally, I was counting on a white knight to save me from my broody, angsty self and maybe even save us all, just like in the movies, books, and television shows I pored over. I've often imagined that this is how young girls get groomed. They just need enough anger, daddy issues, and *freedom* to be swayed by the flattery and attention. And groomers aren't always seedy pimp types, a la the Lifetime Movie Channel. Sometimes they're just slightly older guys who use their age as power over much younger, less wise girls. That's how it happened for me. I don't even think it would've been immediately recognized as such back then, but as Maya Angelou notably said, (paraphrasing) " ... when you know better, do better." Now I know, and I'm calling it as it was.

At the height of my rebellion, after the second (and, to my knowledge, last) time my stepdad (officially by then) hit my mom, I'd had enough. I regularly challenged him, cussed at him, and antagonized him every chance I got. My later therapist would enlighten me that it was my way of trying to control the chaos and simultaneously protect my family by directing his anger toward me instead. As a result, I'd picked myself up off the floor from his backhand more than once. Meanwhile, I began "dating" a much older guy, lying to my parents about his age. He made me feel seen in a way I didn't at home, and yet also like I was *lucky* someone like him would even give me the time of day. He was sneakier with his abuse because it masqueraded as affection, like how he'd tell me I was a clueless young girl who was just pretty enough to be taken advantage of by creepy guys. *So I'm kinda cute, but stupid. Gee, thanks.* He'd follow that up by telling me how he'd protect me because he loved me, subtly creating a dependence on him. Right about the time I was catching on to his bullshit and attempting to free myself from this obsessive, all-consuming *relationship*, my stepdad literally threw me and my sister out of *his* house.

I came home late one night from another dramatic scene with the groomer asshole. This one might've been the one about how if I wasn't going to have sex with him, then I could just "go home to Mommy." Heading up the walkway to our front door, I heard the stepdad asshole yelling at my sister through the open screen door. I went into codependent fix-it mode (and maybe a little bit of projection mode) and set out to divert his attention. And maybe I could take out my anger with the groomer asshole on him while I was at it—a subconscious two for one.

The screen door was locked, so I shouted over his yelling, "Can you stop yelling long enough to unlock the fucking door and let me in?"

I succeeded. He did in fact come unlock the door and began yelling at me instead of my sister—my ungratefulness, my smart mouth, his house, his rules, and if I didn't like it, I could *get the fuck out*. To which I replied that I would *get the fuck out* if my mom hadn't sold the house my grandfather (my dad's dad) built *for us* to bail him out of his financial mess. And there *was* a financial mess, by the way—something my mom let slip once, which I secretly used as another reason to piss him off. I was good at baiting the hook. The *fish* I caught that night was my whole bedroom being picked up and thrown out onto the front lawn. Then, I was picked up by my neck and pushed through the sidelight window by the front door.

To my mom's credit, she did try to talk him down—unsuccessfully, but she tried. As my feet dangled off the ground and I clawed at his hands, she called the police ... but not really. She called our family cop friend. And while my stepdad no longer worked in law enforcement, he was still *a friend of the badge*. When the cop showed up, not only was my stepdad not in trouble, but *I* was instead, and was ordered to stop being an ungrateful, asshole kid or I'd get arrested. Typing this still makes my heart race—about the stepdad or the cop friend's abuse of power? Flip a coin. I guess "protect and serve" is subjective. I still harbor unresolved resentment over it, although I didn't know it until that cop friend recently wanted to stop by my mom's house for a visit while I happened to be there. I made a hasty excuse as to why I had to leave and got the hell out of there. I watched him pull up in his shiny car with his pretty wife—now retired and *reborn*—as I drove away, heart pounding, hands shaking. I recognized at that moment I still had some work to do. I definitely didn't want to continue to drag that guy and his bag of shit around like it was my shit. I had enough of my own shit. Forgiveness and letting go sometimes happen daily, moment to moment. Repeatedly, until my emotions catch up to my goals for inner peace.

For days after the stepdad incident, I couldn't even talk due to my bruised vocal cords. I could barely look at my mom because she didn't protect me. Luckily, I didn't have to, since I wasn't living there. I couch surfed until I could afford my own place. My heart breaks for that kid, and her mom. To this day, nothing can trigger me more than a kid caught in a bad home situation they can't get out of. But I was out after that. Not by choice, but I wasn't going back. No matter what. That was it. I was a legal adult (barely), and even if I couldn't afford it, I knew I wasn't going back. I quit junior college, got a second job, and found a bug-infested studio apartment I could afford. The cherry on top is that I went back to the *comfort* of the icky, sneakily abusive relationship I'd just found my way out of. The epitome of that saying, "better the devil you know." My mom stayed with hers, so I guess the apple didn't fall far from the role model. Here's another saying: children live what they learn. It would take me two more years to unlearn staying with an asshole man. It would take decades, two fathers' deaths, and a cancer diagnosis (or two) for this to translate to *all* my relationships across the board—friends and stepsisters included, although I didn't see the stepsister thing coming.

When faced with a disease that wants to take over your body and kill you, the deep dives on how to fix it become top priority. At least, they did for me. This is where fixing all the issues in my tissues came into play. Some people get treatment (surgery, chemo, radiation) and call it good. I needed to get to the bottom of how it happened in the first place so it could never happen again. I was the quintessential "but why" kid growing up, and I guess I still was. When only 5 to 10 percent of cancers are genetic, that means 90 to 95 percent are caused by controllable variables. I was hellbent on getting to the bottom of it and taking out the trash. Trauma is a habit. We have to discover it, recognize it, and move through it. Essentially, we need to unlearn it to feel safe and calm inside so our bodies feel supported. A body has the ability to heal itself from so much when it has what it needs to heal. We just need to learn how to give it what it needs.

After the abusive incidents, my mom stayed with my stepdad, so he was always around. I stayed away from them both as much as possible and ignored my mom completely for a short while, but she was my mom and I loved her. And I missed her—and a girl needs her mom. He didn't apologize for his behavior in so many words, but he helped me move into my place and became a genuinely good guy—his version of an apology, I realized. Eventually I forgave him, sort of. I mostly gaslit myself that I deserved it for being a disrespectful, ungrateful kid to a man who didn't have to be my dad. Like, "at least he was there for you. Your real dad wasn't." Ever the romantic GenXer, wanting that storybook life and happily ever after, I bought into the fairytale I so desperately wanted. And we made some great memories as a happy family over the years. He adored my husband, rarely missed a chance to watch my kids' games, and was a solid presence and support in my life. But there is also that saying that leopards don't change their spots. Although we got along famously, with many pictures of family trips to prove it, I can look back and see that I still tiptoed around him, like I knew I had a dog that could turn on me at any moment.

When I told him I was writing a book—my very first published book, *Chemo Pissed Me Off*—after a lifetime of dreaming about it, he didn't say "good for you" or "congratulations" or "I'm proud of you." He said, "leave me out of it." I was much older now and frankly, after surviving my own cancer diagnosis, I was beyond tiptoeing around him. Sort of. I didn't yell at him; I yelled at my mom instead. I think I said, "Fine, can you put my mom on the phone?" Utterly fuming on the inside with the years of bullshit I'd put up with, I told her that I'd been through enough of his shit over the years and gone to enough therapy and done enough soul-searching. I wasn't going to allow his toxic shit in my life anymore. I certainly wasn't going to stand for it to be modeled for my kids. And, finally, that if he wanted to be in my life at all, he'd better knock it off and get his shit together.

He ended up apologizing, to my *husband*, "for pissing off your wife." That's some next-level misogynistic shit! I can't even wrap my brain around it to this day! But out of respect for him, I did leave him out of it. But also, for better or worse, this is not that book. And in the spirit of dealing with the issues in my tissues, I'm done gaslighting myself and everyone else and sugarcoating my life. I don't hate him. I love him. I'm grateful for his presence in my life. I am. But as I said, it's a mixed bag.

I'm just going to rip the bandage off here. Somewhere in the middle of my reconstruction waiting game, my stepdad got diagnosed with Stage 4 lung cancer. When I got the news, I saw the writing on the wall. I began sobbing on the phone to my favorite stepsister. We'd grown close in our adult, married, young-parenthood phase of life. She was arguably *my person*. Our families vacationed together, Christmas-ed together, and she and I talked regularly. We'd understandably had a few ups and downs over the years (nothing is perfect), but mostly I thought we were solid. Wrong!

When I called her upon hearing his diagnosis, I didn't really get the reaction I thought I would. She sounded mostly like she was trying to calm an irrational child. In hindsight, I've often wondered if she was experiencing her own triggered trauma response to his diagnosis and just didn't have it in her to deal with mine. Not that I was trying to lay it all on her—I was simply reaching out to *my person*. But I quickly remembered that she wasn't on my level with cancer awareness. She'd never been on my level of questioning doctors, diets, lifestyles, and getting to the *why* of things. She was with the masses in the camp of cancer being the luck of the draw, and had said as much over the years.

I've said many times that I wouldn't wish cancer on anyone, but the perspective from this side is nice. This is not to say I'd want anyone to *get* cancer. Please know that! I'd just seen a lot of cancer situations in the over thirteen years of my own ordeal. It's the club no one wants to be in, but once you're in it, you're in it. You meet others in the club and hear their stories, *for-ev-er* (she said, in the voice of Squints from *The Sandlot*). For me, it has helped me prioritize my life better, not waste my moments as much, or take as many things for granted. Like I said, the perspective is nice, even if the gained insight and knowledge came by way of a scary diagnosis.

Stage 4 folks are in an uphill battle. Every single one of them. Many are referred to hospice care upon getting the diagnosis or told to get their affairs in order. For those who may not know, hospice care focuses on the care, comfort, and quality of life of a person with a serious illness who is approaching the end of their life. I'd seen some incredible cases of radical remission and people surviving and thriving despite a Stage 4 diagnosis, but those cases were rare, with most of those individuals radically changing their lifestyles and belief systems. I knew this was the beginning of the end for him. I sobbed to her on the phone for everything I saw rolling out over the next six to nine months, which is what statistics gave him with his diagnosis.

Her response: "We're not there yet."

That's it! The equivalent of "you need to calm down." She wasn't mean or rude about it, but it was clear the conversation was closed for discussion. I quickly reeled it back. I think that's the moment things changed between us—or that's when I noticed it. Looking back, I think she may have been done with me long before that. Maybe this just gave her the out she needed. I began recalling every weird thing she'd said to me in our recent past that I'd glazed over at the time, and how our relationship had changed and now felt like work.

I'd flashback to small comments she'd made alluding to obligatory visits like I'd become a chore, part of her to-do list. With my newfound perspective, that's pretty far from what I'm about. If having a legitimate relationship with me is a *job*, then don't have one. And that sounds spiteful, but underneath the pain, I meant it in a greater good kind of way. Life is too short for relationships that masquerade as work. I'm human. It sucks to feel rejected or like someone doesn't want you anymore. There was a whole lot of *what the hell happened*. But, perspective ... go in love and Godspeed! But it took my heart a minute to catch up with my mind.

Just recently, I've realized some things about the way my brain works that can be challenging for the people who love me. I likely have undiagnosed ADHD, but I can't say for sure. *One issue at a time!* One night, after another epiphany on my road of growth, I turned to my husband and, choking up a little in the delivery, said, "Maybe if she'd known this about my brain, she wouldn't have thrown me away."

He reminded me of my own words. "What do you always say? When people show you who they are, believe them. You're better off without her in your life." He said other things too, nice things, like how he's sure we're both probably happier now, and things like that. All the stuff I knew, and know. Sometimes it helps to hear someone else say it out loud.

At first, my eighty-two-year-old stepdad said he would change things and wanted to "beat this thing." I readily accommodated, updating him on all I'd learned. He read all the books I brought him about healing Stage

4 cancer and tried to change his diet. The reality was that he was the proverbial old dog who wasn't so keen on learning new tricks. He turned eighty-three under hospice care at home and died three months later, six months after his diagnosis. I was grateful he didn't have long to suffer and that my mom didn't have to watch him fade away for very long. She would say repeatedly toward the end, "It's like he's given up." I don't know if it was that so much as he was losing the race against the prolific cancer cells. Either way, it was heartbreaking. My own ordeal made it easier for me to step back from his situation and not take on the fix-it role I'd claimed most of my life—as much as I wish we could *fix* every cancer diagnosis. I obviously helped where I could, while keeping my own health front and center, but it felt like too little too late. I felt weirdly detached as I watched it all unfold.

My stepdad was a man who didn't sit still much. He'd actively lived almost every ounce of his eighty-three years on earth—even more than we realized. After his death, my mom, my sister and I found out that his longtime, *current* girlfriend died of breast cancer two years before him. That's also when we found out that he *had* a current girlfriend in the first place. The *love of his life*, according to one card we found. That discovery triggered a memory of my stepdad showing up at my house unannounced one day, two years-ish prior, *just to hang out*. I also recalled how he emotionally told us (my husband and me) that he'd lost a *close friend* to cancer that day and just needed to get out of the house. It is not lost on me that he came to my house. He did say he tried to call my stepsister, but she was busy.

I'm just going to say it. I think I was his favorite.

Maybe because I stood up to him and challenged him. Maybe because my husband and my kids played his two favorite sports and he related to them more. But either way, he went out of his way to be part of my adult life and my family's life, more so than I saw him attempting to with his own kids and grandkids. I'm also just going to say this: I was glad he was gone, but not in a malicious way. I'm grateful that his suffering was short. I can't explain the immediate relief I felt when he was gone, but I've sure thought a lot about why that was my first reaction. He was such a force in life, I hated to see him withering away. I was beyond grateful it didn't last long. But I also felt free, and like my mom was free. In the weeks and months after his death, when it would just be the three of us (my mom, my sister, and me) cleaning out his stuff, there was an ease, a simplicity. No one criticizing my mom, her speaking freely without stuttering, a collective exhale of breath I didn't even realize we were all holding.

I vividly remember getting the call:

"Mom, mom." My youngest daughter's distress startled me awake. Nothing can pierce a mother's sleep like the sound of her child's voice. She burst through my bedroom door and all I could see was the light from her phone coming at me in the dark.

"He's dead," she sobbed, pushing her phone to my ear.

Grabbing the phone, I said, "Mom? I'm on my way."

Though I'd had my phone lying right by my head for weeks now anticipating the call—turned up, even—I missed her call. My daughter, home visiting from college, got the call instead.

Relief! Even in my groggy-from-sleep state, I remember that overwhelming feeling. I was relieved that the worst of it lasted only months, for everyone's sake, but mostly his. The man I visited over the last two months wasn't my stepdad, anyway. Instead, it was the shell of a man riddled with cancer, deteriorating before my eyes. He resembled the stepdad I grew up with, the ever-present grandpa at most of my kids' games—just an emaciated, older, weaker version. I'm not sure it was okay to feel that way, but I was relieved.

When I walked into my mom's house, my sister was already there, as she lived the closest. Shortly after, both stepsisters arrived separately. My sister was quick to hug each of them and tell them she was sorry. I hugged them also but didn't say anything. The energy coming off them was tangible, and weird. After years of my deep dives into energy and healing, I was more aware of it now than ever. Death in a room is a crazy, palpable thing. Most people aren't great at handling death to begin with, but this seemed like something more than sorrow. Like coiled wire waiting to spring loose.

After the coroner and hospice left and my stepdad was taken, my mom and stepsisters began discussing logistics, who to call, etc. I felt led to stay out of it as clearly as if the request had been spoken aloud. Until one point, when the eldest stepsister suggested she take her dad's phone with her to contact people for my mom.

My mom gave a tentative, "Okay," as she looked up, making eye contact with me.

I could see on her face that she wasn't *okay* with that. And so, with decades of being the designated pit bull of the family, I took a deep breath and said,

"Maybe we could just get the numbers off of it for you instead of you taking the phone."

I swear on everything I believe that I said it just like that. No sass or animosity. If anything, I was overly nice.

She countered with all the venom of her own issues— which she'd evidently kept just under the surface all these years. "That is why I asked the question *to your mother*, and she *agreed.*"

I wish I could accurately convey how hateful she sounded. She spewed the words through clenched teeth without raising her voice, and seemed to ooze hatred. I wish I was just being dramatic here. It was creepy. My heart began to pound as I calmly tried to explain that my mom experienced forty years of not speaking up for herself, being married to an abusive man—and that's when she jumped up, grabbed her things and started saying she wasn't going to listen to this and began to storm out. As she did, her sister, *my person*, followed suit without saying a word. It's like they'd rehearsed what to do if they got pissed off or offended.

Hindsight: terrible choice of words. I began backpedaling, trying to get them to stay. I'm not even sure what I said. I tend to do this people-pleasing, fast-talking thing when I'm nervous or in socially awkward situations. When nothing I said worked and only prompted more venomous shots from the eldest, I think I spouted something sarcastic like, "Great way to handle this." I honestly don't recall, but it sounds like something I'd say.

On her way out the door, the youngest barked in defense of her sister, "She just lost her father."

To which I quickly hurled, "So did I." *Why is she excused from being an asshole over her grief, but I am not?*

She barked back, "Oh, you always have to make everything about you."

Stunned into silence, I watched them walk out. My mom followed them out to try to ... I don't know, fix it?! I sat frozen, mind reeling, not knowing what to say or do, but the old tapes played a familiar tune in my head: *it's all your fault, you do and say all the wrong things, you fuck everything up, (and, a new one:) they think you make everything about you—and always have.* And that last little fucked-up narrative lived rent free in my head for months to come—while I went through reconstruction surgeries and quite literally fought for my life. No wonder that first surgery went so horribly wrong. My tissues were full of issues. But back to that night ...

As my sister, husband, and I sat in the charged silence of their storming out, my husband pierced the quiet with levity as he can so readily do—humor being his defense mechanism against his own shitty stepfather and GenX neglect. "Well, that didn't take long. Who had twenty minutes?"

My sister laughed out loud and they both began *trying* to make light of the situation. It's worth noting that my husband doesn't hate anyone. Not even his own abusive ex-stepfather. And equally, most people absolutely adore him. He's easy to like. He gets along with anyone and everyone, but can barely tolerate my eldest stepsister and has even used the words "I can't stand her." He's said he's never seen anyone change the energy of a room like she can, and not in a good way. While he and my sister tried to lighten things up, I continued to play the old tapes in my head, barely listening to their banter. *I make everything worse. I say the wrong things. I don't think before I speak. I'm difficult. It's all my fault. Nobody gets me. They don't love me. I'm unlovable.* And the new tape courtesy of my stepsister: *I guess I make everything about me. Do I? I don't think that's true. I just try to fix things. But she believes that, and clearly always has. My dad just died, and this is what I'm thinking about. Maybe I do make everything about me. Otherwise, I wouldn't be sitting here thinking about this. I just want everything to be okay. How do I do that?*

For the record, I've come a long way from that person who believed those tapes. But when something catastrophic happens, it's incredibly easy to throw them back in and press play. It's unconscious. I slipped back into that codependent fixer in crisis mode. I hate that! I love that girl, but I hate her MO. I like the new girl who can stop and take a breath and calmly assess what's really going on. The one who doesn't fast-talk her way through shit to make everyone else feel better, while ignoring her own pain.

When my mom didn't return more than fifteen minutes later, I, still in crisis mode, decided to go out and check on her, maybe attempt at damage control— ever the fixer. I found the three of them still talking in the driveway.

I approached and said, "I do not have to be a part of any of this, if that would make it easier for you guys. I want you guys to get what you need out of this. I do not need the rituals to make my peace with his passing."

And that was true. I secretly disliked cemeteries and funerals. The person I lost was no longer here on this earth and going to a plot of ground to pay my respects did not bring me closer to my loved one or give me any peace. I don't mind the receptions, where everyone is sharing memories and there is fellowship. Mostly though, I think we do a terrible job of processing death in western cultures. To each his own. I'm just saying I don't need the rituals. My mom spoke up and said she wanted me to be part of things. The steps agreed, and eventually came back inside to finalize a game plan of what would come next.

After some semblance of civility, the eldest surprisingly hugged me as she left and mumbled something nice like, "It's a hard time for everyone." A valid attempt at forgiveness to my way of thinking and very big of her, considering how pissed off she clearly still was. After she left, the youngest sat with me and *tried* to talk through *our* shit, but she brought up years-old arguments, disagreements, things I didn't even know still bothered her and things that I never knew did, that she was clearly not over. Fun fact about me is I can get extremely heated in the moment. I've learned that people with ADHD have impulse control issues, especially when angry. I've always known I had anger issues, but only recently learning possibly why. Still, when things have calmed down and conversations of forgiveness have taken place, it's done for me. So, while I was treating our relationship the same as ever, she was apparently storing up wrongs I'd done and weighing which would be the proverbial straw that broke the camel's back. Maybe not, but that's how it was shaping up for me in that space.

During our conversation, none of my therapy talk worked. Making "I" statements, no "you" statements, actively listening, mirroring her body language, all ricocheted off her futilely. They ironically seemed to upset her more. Maybe my "I" statements just reinforced that *I make everything about me.* Like I said, that damn narrative had set up camp in my brain. Another thing she said at the end of our conversation that staked its claim in my head was, "I just need to think about this."

To this day, I don't know what that means. Think about what? Whether I "passed" the test of our conversation? Whether she can still be my friend, my family, in my life? Whether she can ever admit that she isn't always right? Whether she can believe I'm not the narcissist she has decided I am? Whether she deserves a seat at the table of my life? Whatever it was, she is apparently still thinking about it. While we did have a few text conversations about the funeral arrangements, I haven't seen her since that night. As of the writing of this, it's been two years. We sent check-in, birthday and holiday texts back and forth for a while, but eventually those stopped too. My very last text to her was: *Hopefully we can catch up soon.* It was met with crickets, and I haven't heard from her since.

My birthday would've been the next obligatory holiday text and ... there was nothing. So, when hers came around, I followed suit. And not in a tit-for-tat kind of way. For me, it's a reciprocity thing. One-sided relationships are a ridiculous waste of time and energy. My relationship judgment is admittedly impaired by my childhood baggage. But throughout this cancer journey, I've been committed to *taking out the trash*. I put things, especially relationships, through the filter of codependency, recognize the toxic traits, and attempt to rectify or release them. I recognize that as I no longer tolerate my dysfunctional default setting, some of my old habits and past relationships will not survive. Still, some of the people and things that end up on the cutting room floor surprise me. Some, not at all.

My eldest stepsister wouldn't even communicate with me via text after my stepdad died. During the planning of the funeral, she sent messages through my mom. So much for that forgiveness hug goodbye. I felt completely uninvited to their inner circle of family and was not about to assume any roles or "make anything about me." I offered to make programs. I got the younger's approval on the rough draft and ordered them. They showed up glossy instead of matte. I tried to fix it but ran out of time. In the end, we had glossy programs—which I just knew was another strike against me. I knew I'd fallen short—again. My stepdad would not have given one shit about the finish on his programs—a small thing that brought me solace. Besides, I had bigger fish to fry. I was finally getting my surgery and not even a funeral could stop me.

Maybe I did make everything about me. But the funeral timeline wasn't mine and neither was the surgery timeline. So *did* I? Also, if I truly was the self-centered, make-everything-about-me narcissist she decided I was, would I even be wondering this or concerned at all? And in the spirit of *not* vilifying either of them, perhaps when relationships stop bringing out the best in us and start feeling like a job, maybe losing them is a blessing in disguise for everyone. No hero. No villain. Just growth.

Yeah, let's go with that. Because when the hospital called to cancel my original surgery date, I had two options: take the date they had coming up in just two weeks and miss the funeral, or wait another three months. I took what I considered *my* blessing in disguise.

Chapter 7

The Big Bad Surgery
and the One After That

Courage is the resistance to fear, mastery of fear –
not the absence of fear.
~Mark Twain

From that initial meeting with the first *rockstar*, a cardiologist dedicated to lymphatic research, I was finally getting the surgery with his equally rockstar-esque plastic microsurgeon eight months later. There was no way I was putting it off any longer, funeral or no funeral. Besides, I didn't need the rituals, remember? And the rockstar title cannot be overstated for either of them. He is highly educated and has been the founder of more research and education than I will even try to list here. He has also sufficiently made history and secured his spot in the books, trust me on this.

Eight months earlier, when I finally got in to see him via video visit, he deemed I was more than qualified to move onto the next level—seeing his appointed plastic surgeon who specializes in lymph node transplants. She had equally attained rockstar status, unbeknownst to me at the time. Again, there was more waiting. Since one in eight women get breast cancer, I was not the only one seeking this treatment—not even close.

Just to recap that initial appointment with the rockstar plastic surgeon ...

What I understood the surgery to entail versus what would happen were worlds apart. Here's the thing about surgeons—most that I've met anyway—they aren't so big on the patient care aspect of things. They're big on the intricacies of what they do. In this case, this surgeon was a microsurgeon and essentially a standalone in her field. She, and the nurse before her, came in talking about how she would remove my abdomen skin and fat and pull it down tight, resulting in a tummy tuck, and then use that skin to make boobs. I know! This description is always met with the oohs and ahhs of "lucky," "I'd love a tummy tuck," and my personal favorite, "I have extra fat you can use if you want." To which I'd reply, "I wish." And I kind of did. Whether I had enough fat to make enough breasts to be *breasts* remained to be seen.

This is a lovely little side benefit for our middle aged, child-born bellies—in theory. Believe me when I say, it's not all it's cracked up to be, and this *side benefit* pales in comparison to the reality of the actual ordeal. I've done some electively painful things in the name of beauty, like laser hair removal, for example. Painful as hell, but I don't regret it for a second. And the beauty part of hair removal was frankly just the cherry on top. It was more about the ease of planning outfits and not having to shave every day. Anyone with a five o'clock armpit shadow feels me on this. I'd say it was more about efficiency or, if I'm being honest, laziness. And that "no hair" thing came in handy when I was stuck in a hospital bed for five days straight—*twice*! At one point, a nurse even commented on how I had no armpit hair. I immediately envisioned days of armpit hair growth and the smells that inevitably came with it, and felt sympathy for the nurses wading through all that—and patients who had to suffer that indignity on top of the many others that come with lengthy hospital stays and immobility. But I digress.

I had been referred to this plastic surgeon in the first place for a lymph node transplant, which I would get in my left arm to hopefully stop any swelling from lymphedema along with breast reconstruction. My left breast implant had developed contracture (tightening and distortion of the implant, causing it to shift upward on the chest wall) due to radiation treatments, which meant I'd need more than just the lymph node transplant. I needed a new boob job, too. The first step to that is an explant surgery to remove the implants and the scar tissue around them. There is also the real issue of post-cancer patients being conscious of their immune systems, remember? And any foreign objects in your body can create an immune response that runs quietly in the background. In simple terms, it means your immune system could allow an environment where cancer cells fly under the radar undetected. This is the very nature of a cancer cell. It mimics a healthy cell just enough to slip by the *guards*, a.k.a. the immune system. Making sure your immune system isn't constantly distracted by *shiny objects* like implants can be highly beneficial for a post-cancer treatment system like mine. So, I began looking into alternatives. To me, all the options sounded barbaric. But DIEP flaps, as mine are called, made the most sense to me. Although getting the procedure done absolutely freaked me out.

A DIEP (pronounced *deep*) flap is a type of reconstruction surgery that uses a woman's own abdominal tissue to create a new breast after a mastectomy. The name comes from branches of the primary blood vessel relocated during the procedure, the deep inferior epigastric perforator (DIEP). In a DIEP flap, fat, skin, and blood vessels are cut from the wall of the lower belly and moved up to the chest to rebuild the breast.

The surgeon's nurse explained that each flap can take four to five hours to complete in surgery, which included removing tissue, preparing tissue, and then attaching it along with the blood vessels. They'd place my omentum tissue (more on that in a moment) in my upper left arm to provide a working lymph system. She further explained that it would require a four to five-day hospital stay. And for some reason, this was the scariest part for me. The "pulling off" of my skin freaked me out, yes, but I had no frame of reference for the actuality of it. Hospitals? I don't like them. At this point, I told the nurse that the tummy tuck part wasn't what I understood the procedure to be, and that I wanted to discuss other options. She tried to talk me down, so to speak, but I dug my heels in and wouldn't budge. Wrestling my panic, I asked to talk to the surgeon. I'd envisioned outpatient surgery, which is what all my others had been. But this was major surgery with multiple things happening in one event. I was scared.

When the surgeon came in, she reiterated what the nurse already told me, but she said we could try an omental flap surgery. In simple terms, omentum is a deep layer of fat that lays over our abdominal organs. Technically, it is a large, flat, adipose tissue layer nestling on the surface of the intraperitoneal organs (liver, spleen, stomach, and parts of the colon). Besides fat storage, omentum has key biological functions in immune regulation and tissue regeneration.

In technical terms, omentum biological properties include neovascularization, haemostasis, tissue healing and regeneration, and as an *in vivo* incubator for cells and tissue cultivation. Again, in simple terms, the omentum is great for live boobs because it is vascular. It has veins, arteries, and lymph nodes. It can also be removed laparoscopically, which is less invasive than the DIEP flap procedure. But this would delay my procedure because a general surgeon would need to assist, as they are the ones removing the omentum for the plastic surgeon to use. It required the meshing of three separate schedules: the OR, the plastic, and the general. I waited months.

I had no idea just how highly sought-after my rockstar plastic *micro* surgeon was. When I finally got my number called, I was back in the surgeon's office discussing how the procedure would go. She informed me that there was a great likelihood I would not have enough omentum to even make two boobs. That I could very likely wake up almost flat chested after going through the procedure, or even slightly concave. A peculiar fun fact about omentum and how much each person has: there is no way to know until you physically get in there and take it. It has nothing to do with a person's size or weight. *Why couldn't she have just said all that two months ago?*

In that new pre-op discussion, we went back to the first option: the tummy tuck DIEP flap. My husband and I agreed that it would be the best option, although it sounded barbaric as hell and scared the shit out of me. The hospital stay alone alarmed me enough to consider foregoing it all. I'd contemplated living with what I thought would be an athletic-looking flat chest. But after removing implants, I'd have the saggy skin the implants had stretched and two concave holes where boobs were supposed to be. That wasn't a look I was prepared to live with. Now we were back to square one with this surgeon, a few months further down the road with a few more to go for her availability. Seriously, why couldn't she just have explained all that a few months prior? I still don't know, but I'm a believer in timing and divine intervention, so I'm trusting this was *meant to be.*

I was having three flaps done: two breasts via tummy tuck and one lymph node transplant via omentum, which would go on the inside of my left bicep, just above my elbow. Not to mention the explant before that to clear the space for the new boobs. She said the surgery would take about nine hours, but it ended up taking fifteen! During the last five hours, my husband and entire support system were on pins and needles, wondering what the hell was taking so long. It was after the surgery that we got to know that each flap routinely took four to five hours. Why didn't she just say that to begin with?

This is where that "lack of surgeon bedside manner" thing comes in. Not one to mince words, I asked in post op why she didn't just tell us it would take fourteen to fifteen hours instead of worrying everyone. She gave a vague answer about logistics and booking ORs and general bureaucracy that didn't quite answer the question. I pushed further, wanting to know what happened in that surgery. It seemed like she was hiding something—because, let's face it, things didn't go as we'd hoped or planned. And it's occurred to me more than once that maybe they purposely disclose as little as possible so we won't get horrified enough to cease being their human guinea pigs. I'm willing to concede that this may be my mere mortal brain not understanding the intricacies of the human body and medical intervention, but again, I digress. Five *extra* hours in the OR while everyone you love is flipping out seems easily avoidable with a little communication. The texts my husband did get were things like "everything is going well" and other equally uninformative generalizations. Again, maybe I don't get it, but it seems simple enough to just do better. Say more. Explain. I think the biggest culprit was the bureaucracy of scheduling surgeries. I'm going to lay down my conspiracy theory sword and go with that.

I missed my stepdad's funeral for this surgery. It's true I didn't care about burial rituals, but I would have loved to have been there for my mom. In hindsight, I highly recommend handling your trauma baggage before heading into a major surgery or anything that requires immense physical healing. Being fully present for the healing task at hand cannot be overstated. Remember, the issues are in the tissues. Our bodies physically process unresolved emotional trauma in stress, pain, and disease. My available bandwidth was not sufficient for processing this family trauma, although I gave it a valiant effort. I did all the things: I journaled about it, prayed about it, and spoke words of forgiveness and blessings over my step family and myself daily, sometimes hourly. I did all the self-talk affirmations about how what people think or believe about me is none of my business and not about me anyway. I practiced gratefulness in *all* things like my life depended on it. And didn't it? But these things take time, much more than the two weeks I had before surgery. As I said, the surgery didn't go exactly as planned or even remotely close to how we'd hoped.

It's worth mentioning that the surgery waiting game isn't just about sitting around waiting for the call. I also had a semi-love/hate relationship with this rockstar surgeon. She was undeniably good at what she did and was highly sought after but the last-minute cancellations and reschedules were frankly a pain in the ass for everyone involved and a stressor I didn't need. Just the juggling alone was a serious commitment to boobs. When the call came in, it was a mad shuffle of events and schedules for more than just me. I don't think that's how most surgeries go. But this seemed standard protocol for this surgeon. It happened more than it didn't–at least to me.

As a last hurrah of sorts before I would be on a three-month recovery grind (well before the rescheduling drama), we had planned to meet our best friends for a quick couples' weekend getaway just before the original surgery date. When the surgery got moved up, instead of canceling entirely, we encouraged our guys to keep the date (roughly two weeks after my new surgery date) and just have a guy trip. Meanwhile, *my girl* would come for a staycation with me, sunning by the pool and checking up on me while I pretty much held my bed down to the floor. I'd been through surgery before, and my body mostly handled it like a champ. I thought, win-win. We sorely underestimated the grind of this surgery *and* the recovery. In hindsight, my previous experiences with surgery were quick, usually outpatient. This was the opposite of that.

When I woke up in the hospital fourteen hours later, I can't say that I knew something was wrong. I can say that I'd never felt like that after a surgery. Groggy is a gross understatement. I felt drugged. I imagine it's what being roofied would feel like. You know how on screen the camera sways and spins to make the audience *feel* what the character is going through? Like that! I had no idea I'd been under for fourteen hours. I woke up in a huge, dark, private room in the middle of the night, alone, head swimming, with lots of bandages and multiple abandoned IV sites. There were two male nurses hovering around me, speaking calmly and slowly. Within a couple hours, I was moved from my private palace into a cramped, brighter room with a roommate. I remember them saying they needed the private room for a contagious patient. Not that I cared as my head swam and I fought to grasp my situation. I was alone and in survival mode. And when I say cramped, I'm not being a dramatic, entitled diva. Doctors and nurses were literally tripping over each other and the equipment to tend to me, butt-bumping each other and fumbling things, apologizing to each other as they went. And for me, it was all happening in hasty slow motion.

The first twenty-four hours after this type of live tissue surgery, nurses and doctors come in every hour to check for a doppler signal of connected veins and arteries. At first they couldn't find the doppler machine, so they launched into panic mode, running around and checking different wards before they located one. And this machine was an obnoxious little box! Once turned on, it would make a constant, ear-splitting static until it found a heartbeat. When it did find one, it would begin to thump like an ultrasound machine relaying a baby's heartbeat. While this chaos ensued, the nurses and doctors flooded me with a barrage of questions every hour, asking my name, birthdate, and why I was there. Standard operating procedure in the medical world, I know, but it just added another layer to the chaos. And it was happening at a teaching hospital, so there was a constant crew of people with clipboards taking notes and/or asking questions. At times there were pop-quiz questions for the "learners."

Another fun fact of DIEP flap with a lymph node transplant is the need for what they call the BAIR hugger for the first two to three days. It's a heated, paper-like blanket that blows warm or hot air on the flaps to assist in blood circulation of the reconstructed area. It feels extremely warm and is known to cause restlessness. *No shit!* If they didn't tuck that blanket around me just right, the hot air would blow onto my face and make me feel like I couldn't breathe. I had more than one panic attack over the BAIR hugger situation. *Good times!* It's ridiculous to me that they stress the intense recovery required for these surgeries (restful, peaceful, etc.) and the first five days in the hospital are anything but. It's loud, bright, chaotic, and just for fun, let's throw in the indignity of needing help with everything, including taking a sip of water and wiping your butt. I won't even get into the restricted use of my arms, but I resembled a

T-rex. *For weeks!* I know, you're wondering again why I bothered. I have asked myself this too many times. I wanted boobs. I still do. I wanted a chest that felt and looked normal(ish). I wanted a calm immune system. I wanted to hopefully undo everything cancer, chemo, and radiation had done to my body.

During the five-day hospital stay, I developed a significant hematoma in my right boob and required a blood transfusion. That explained the drugged feeling—internal bleeding. The nurses and doctors kept telling me I'd feel so much better after the transfusion. I kept waiting for the better to come, and I guess I did feel marginally better right after and got some color back, but I wasn't grading on a curve. I still felt like a roofied co-ed and when I said I was pale, I mean I almost matched the sheets. The color I got back from the infusion didn't last. I looked like death and didn't feel much better.

Within the first twenty-four hours of surgery, they wanted me to get up and walk around. I warned them that I was dizzy and could barely stand on my own and make it to the bathroom without help. I wanted to be tough and kept telling myself that I should feel better than I did. The nurses kept harping on me to get up and move around—nicely, but they were insistent. I'm good at following directions, so I walked up and down the hall with a walker and a helper by my side, because they didn't trust me not to fall. I kept asking her why I felt so dizzy, even after the blood transfusion. Though I felt marginally better, I still needed help and I couldn't understand why. I wanted answers and they didn't seem to have any. They were still getting a doppler signal from each flap, including the one with the ginormous hematoma. So, they released me on schedule after five days. I wanted to go home, thinking maybe that's what I needed to finally feel better. I still hadn't regained my color or equilibrium. The right boob swelling was inexplicable. The three-hour drive home was damn near unbearable. The last hour of the drive I spent writhing in pain, involuntary tears leaking down my face. So much for peaceful relaxation.

All three hospital stays throughout my reconstruction were nightmarish. I'm not being dramatic for effect here. I'm not sure anyone likes hospitals, but my three recent stays are even hard to recount for the sake of this book. The first one was pretty bad and I'm not even sure it was the worst. My right arm had so much edema post-surgery that the hospital bands were indenting my wrist. You know those loose paper bands? Yeah, they were bursting at the seams, so to speak. Running antibiotics and pain medication through my IV was excruciating. I remember crying silently in pain as one nurse administered it. I pleaded with him to let me take it orally. He immediately asked the rockstar, who said no, because IV was safer. She was concerned about infection. So, he came back and proceeded, despite my obvious pain. He rubbed my hand as he did it, apologizing over and over.

The next time around, a different nurse came in. And before she got started, I told her how bad it hurt and again asked for oral medication. She explained that the doctor wanted IV because they're more effective, and she didn't want to run the risk of infection. *Yeah, I know.* As the medication hit my veins, the searing pain caused me to yelp. I tried to rein it in, but the pain was too much. Not to sound like a song lyric, but it felt like fire in my veins. By the way, if I haven't mentioned it, this is all because I chose to do my four rounds of chemo through an IV instead of a port. It basically turned my veins to concrete, according to numerous medical staff who've experienced my IV issues firsthand. *Who knew?* After a very long few seconds of the IV drugs and me crying through the pain, she said, "Okay, that's it."

I think I heard her utter the F-word under her breath, too. I can't be sure. I was a bit incoherent at that time, but her body language was clear. Her Hippocratic oath was intact, and she would not be subjecting me to this torture any longer. I didn't get the bitchy vibe from her. On the contrary, I got the "I'm advocating for this patient" vibe.

She said, "I'm getting you the oral medication." *My hero!*

And just to further paint the picture of this freak show, at one point, my hospital roommate asked if I'd been in a car accident as she walked past my bed to get to the restroom. In other words, *damn girl, you look like shit*. Between the dizziness, paleness, the painful IV, having to get help for everything from peeing to lifting a water pitcher, and let's not forget looking like I'd been in a car accident apparently, there was *no* peace. I still don't know how I could've been expected to rest, recover, or stay calm. I was constantly talking myself down from panic, except during the moments of fitful, drug-induced sleep. And did I mention the hives? My entire torso was covered in them. From the pre-surgery wash? The adhesive? The surgical tape? The sutures? No one knows. But I was covered in those itchy little jerks. I just wanted to go home. And why does it take them hours to discharge you once you finally get the greenlight to go home? Every single time!

At ten days post-surgery, at my follow-up appointment, I explained I was still quite light-headed, although not to the degree I'd been. I still had a swollen but semi-normal looking boob on the left (ironically, the cancer side that had withstood all the treatment), a left bicep that looked (and felt) like it had a small boulder underneath the skin (lymph node transplant), and one enormous freak show of a black, blue, and purple boob on the right that looked like some Academy Award-winning special effect. It was hideous. In doctor speak, it was a hematoma that was slowly resolving.

"Everything is still alive and moving in the right direction," they said. *Oh good, because I was expecting an alien to explode out of that thing at any moment.*

We came home from that visit encouraged, despite the boob FX. We kept tentative plans to go ahead with the modified couples' weekend. My husband had been by my side constantly, doing literally everything for me and continuing to work (remotely, thank God). I wanted him to take the weekend and blow off some steam with his lifelong best buddy. My girlfriend, his wife, assured me she could handle my "gross" boob and was happy to have a lazy girls' weekend in the sun. She's the mom of a lot of boys, so a weekend of chick flicks and lounging by the pool sounded like bliss to her. I was just lucky enough to cash in on that. Again, a win-win, to my way of thinking. Anyone could babysit a patient that was restricted to bed, right?

Not so fast.

Shortly after she arrived, I began feeling extra dizzy again—more than the usual post-surgery dizziness I'd been experiencing. I called the nurse, and she instructed me to head to the emergency department right away. Again, this facility is more than two hours away in good traffic conditions. Why didn't we go to a closer ED? Because if I needed anything, I wanted *my* surgical team to be the ones handling it—the ones who knew all the shit my body had been through. Not some random ED docs in another city. No disrespect, but I was in no condition to give them a rundown and connect the dots.

My gal pal is a trooper. She's from another state and not at all familiar with my area. She called my husband, who was ready to hop in the car and get home (he was three hours away), but she told him she could handle it. Besides, we didn't even know if there was anything *to* handle at that point. He reluctantly agreed. I know some people might judge this, or him, or us right now. Trust me, my guy is an over-the-top husband. I wish I could effectively explain how all my cancer crap had taken its toll on him, and really my whole family. Those who have been through it know. It affects everyone in its path. I wanted this timeout for him and insisted on it, and at the time I couldn't fathom how bad my situation was. I just kept ignorantly expecting everything to work out.

Once we made it to the ED, she dropped me at the door so I wouldn't have to walk from the parking garage—it's a massive place. When I say I could barely walk on my own, I am not exaggerating. I knew something was terribly wrong, but I was in denial about how wrong it really was. Or more likely, I just didn't have the energy or wits about me to sort it all out. I stumbled into the waiting room and was told the ED was at maximum capacity. That meant no one would be allowed in with me. I texted my friend to wait outside for me and found a wall to lean against, ideally away from the *germy* people. Maximum capacity meant there were almost no seats, anyway. There were lots of helpers wading through the crowd, checking in patients as quickly as possible. One such helper took one look at me and streamlined my admittance. I was grateful I looked emergent and not like the junkie I imagined I felt like.

After they got me into a room, it quickly went from "what's going on," to "you're going into surgery." The right flap (boob) had died. I've read conflicting statistics about how often that happens, but generally it's rare. When it does, microsurgery can be performed to reconnect vessels in flaps that are not a total loss. In my case, even if it wasn't a total loss, my rockstar microsurgeon was unavailable. Like, *in another country* unavailable. One of the surgeons on her team performed the surgery, and although also a plastic surgeon specializing in reconstruction, she was not a microsurgeon or a rockstar. No disrespect, just facts. And I know you may be asking, does this microsurgeon even warrant her rockstar nickname? Well, although my surgery went far south from where we'd planned, she is still one of only a couple surgeons that do what she does. I think I heard one of her people say that there is another one in New York, but that's about it. So yeah, rockstar, but even rockstars have a bad show now and then. I was in no state to overanalyze. I was a zombie from bleeding internally and from the flap dying inside my body. All I wanted was relief, and they could provide it. Beyond that, I felt alone. I couldn't have a wingman inside the hospital with me. I couldn't even keep details straight; I was so out of it. It was all just happening and I was along for the ride. I trusted it was their job to keep me alive, but it wasn't a conscious trust. It was more like *sitting-down-in-a-chair* trust. I was doing it. They said encouraging things like, "It may not be dead. We have to get in there and see."

Perhaps my outcome wouldn't have changed even with the rockstar in house. All I know for sure is that I woke up two-and-a-half hours later sans one boob and devastated. I also know from past experiences that tissue needs a minimum of six months to a year to heal before more reconstruction can take place. As it turned out, it was another year, almost to the day, before I got a new boob. One boob and one concave hole where a boob is supposed to be is a far cry from normal. And another year of waiting ... "devastated" is an understatement. I was salty. An incoherent mess of salty sobbing tears. And scars both literal and figurative; and another crappy hospital stay, complete with a heavily perfumed nursing assistant with crazy long nails that invaded my literal personal space.

Why did this make my radar? Because while she was sponging me off, (and don't get me started on that indignity) she transferred her perfume or lotion or whatever the hell it was onto me when lifting and maneuvering me. Did I mention my highly sensitive person status translates to scents, too? And the nails ... yeah. She wiped my *parts* so aggressively, I yelped. She gave a half-ass apology like she didn't think she could have possibly hurt me to the point of a yelp. And she wasn't a jerk. She was nice, super kind even. I can assure you that the absence of hormones changes things down under, and being sensitive is an understatement.

But beyond that, why are you wiping me off like you're changing a shitty diaper? For fuck's sake, I'm a grown ass woman who needed refreshing, not a grownup who'd shit themselves. I was so bothered, I later asked a nurse friend of mine if long nails (and polish) were still not allowed in a hospital setting, because after twenty years of being her friend and seeing her unpolished nails even on dressy occasions, I knew it was a thing. She confirmed it was still not allowed, and said neither was perfume or heavily scented lotions or any strong scents for that matter. She was also shocked by my story, mostly because this happened at a top ten hospital. I am too. It frankly still kind of pisses me off when I think about it. Again, mere mortal here, and not in the business of saving lives and all, but this just seems like common sense to me.

After my two-day, one-night hospital stay, and after I did finally get home (a grueling and painful over-four-hour drive due to the high-traffic time of my discharge), I cried for two days straight. I was under the misconception that they'd taken all my omentum tissue, and I knew they'd taken all my excess belly fat the first time around. The hysteria came from wondering where I'd get enough fat to make another boob to fill the huge boob hole. Turns out, they only took a small amount of omentum for the lymph node transplant and the rest of the omentum would be used later for the fix-it surgery. This is where that "full disclosure" thing comes in handy. And maybe allowing a second set of ears in the room to hear the things you're telling the heavily sedated patient about her procedures. *Remember people, trying to dial down the stress!* I get that the flip side is freaking out the patient with the overshare, but

I'm firmly in the camp of *my body, my decision*. Give me all the information, even when I might later wish for brain bleach to get back my ignorant bliss. It was still too soon to tell if the transplant would stop the lymphedema. I was a swollen black-and-blue mess of recovering flesh. But I was hopeful.

And just so this doesn't become a giant book of complaints, here's a big dose of gratitude for you. I would like to acknowledge how incredibly fortunate I feel to have been pseudo-retired while going through all of this. As cancer diagnoses get younger and younger, I'm hyper-aware of all those going through cancer and cancer treatment who still must work, parent, and run a household. I'm an empty nester, retired, stay-at-home mom-turned-author who can let her housework pile up if she chooses. The blessing and the curse are that while I have plenty of time to do my research and plan anti-cancer diets, workouts, and lifestyle routines, I also have plenty of downtime to obsess, overthink, and worry. This is where therapy would come in handy. The overthinking is real, and paralyzing. Sometimes, the only calming thing I can do is declare a lazy day and binge comfort TV. Rewatching shows for the 100th time is a proven comfort strategy. Not kidding! The psychology behind it is that because we know what's coming, it soothes us. I finally found a soother. You're welcome for the tip, and the greenlight to Netflix and chill—but literally chill, not the Urban Dictionary definition, which is hooking up. My daughters would say that me getting the meaning wrong, intentionally or not, is cringy. But I digress.

My gratefulness truly knows no bounds. It's the reason I wrote my first published book, *Chemo Pissed*

Me Off. It's the reason I'm reliving this reconstruction nightmare on these pages right now. I always say it's not a book I ever thought I'd write, but there I was with all that good material. If it can help someone else get through something like this even a little easier, then I feel like it gives meaning to it all. Helping someone else feel less alone through something like cancer gives me *all the feels*. In fact, check out my cheat sheets of downloadable and printable tips and tricks as my gift to you. Go to www.wylliegirl.com to get yours. You'll find that I try to keep it updated as I learn new things.

But back to the waiting game ...

Chapter 8

The Waiting Game and the Cancellation Queen

" ... we make our plans, and we hear God laughing ...
"

~Thomas Rhett, *Life Changes*

Have you ever heard Christian folks say that whenever you're experiencing extreme impatience, it means you must've prayed for patience and that God is essentially throwing a bunch of things at you that test your patience? First, I don't believe God works that way. And second, I believe we will repeat patterns until we learn the lesson we need to learn. As I said, I believe He can and will use opportunities for our ultimate good, if we're willing. So, patience ...

Ever notice when you're going through something extremely triggering, how the triggers are everywhere? Maybe it's the law of attraction. Over the next year of waiting, I realized I was triggered by TV ads, specifically pharmaceutical ads. And don't get me started on how they find a way to get those ads in our faces, despite our best efforts (in the form of streaming fees) to keep them out. I'd go from zero to setting something on fire within moments. And it doesn't help that the volume increases exponentially when the ad pops up. My point is that even vegging out on TV tested my patience. Every favorite show had a favorite character going through cancer. Even the cop-show violence I used to love set my nerves on edge. And could Nicholas Sparks write one where someone doesn't have a terminal illness and dies?

I also would get a pit in my stomach every time someone told me how great I looked. Weird, right? And I probably did look good ... ish. I spent extra time camouflaging the boob hole and making sure everything else about me looked great because that part of me clearly did not. The epitome of "fake it till you make it," whatever that means. I didn't want to miss my life, but I didn't feel particularly social during my patience testing era. And for those reading this who may have been those people who told me I looked great, please know I love you even more for being *those people* who told me.

It took a few months to snap out of my depression and to physically recover from the back-to-back surgeries. A silver lining is that it put my stepfamily drama on the back burner, out of necessity. An overthinker like me still thought about it, but I didn't obsess about it—much.

When I found out from my husband that my step nephew wouldn't speak to or even acknowledge him at the funeral despite his efforts to be friendly, that put the nail in the coffin for me. Pun not intended. I completely removed the eldest stepsister (his mother) from my life. Follow my reasoning: her son had only her account of what went down the night my stepdad died. And obviously, her version was such that her son was not only pissed on her behalf but was *so* pissed that it spilled over onto my husband who is, as I've said, arguably the nicest person on the planet. And he didn't even *do* anything except be married to me. Even if I didn't have a loyalty streak a mile wide, this would have been enough of an asshole maneuver to get me on board. Gut reaction: she could fuck off forever. But true to my newfound path of peace, I came around to praying for her, genuinely sending her love and light and actively releasing her and my animosity toward her. It was easy to let toxic things go in my state of healing. Life and death has a way of putting things in perspective, and I truly believe we are all better off without relationships that conjure the worst versions of ourselves.

I'm not in the business of hating anyone. Truly! It's a lot of work. Sure there are people in this world I like more than others; that's true for us all. But, I'd much rather spend my time on ... well, almost anything else than on people I don't get along with. And removing her from my life may sound extreme—the grownup equivalent of taking my ball and going home—but I can assure you it's not. I've spent enough time and effort trying to be my best self that I can no longer abide relationships with people who can only see some past version of me, or the worst version of me. Because I know how hard I've had to work to change my own default settings, I can unequivocally recognize that I have no hope of changing someone else's. I can just let them go as peacefully as possible.

My relationship with my other stepsister is a little more complicated. I was much closer to her. Arguably, it was one of my closest female relationships. But it was clear that *ship* had sailed. She didn't check up on me throughout my surgeries or recoveries. I didn't check up on her to see how she was handling her grief. In my defense, I had just come off two horrendous surgeries and was in survival mode. In hers, grief can also feel like survival mode. I'm not competing for who is right here. After almost two years of soul searching, I've decided that God and the universe both recognized that our relationship no longer served either of us. That's about as *zen* as I can be about it.

Part of me wonders if she knew all along about the other woman (or women) and didn't want to face me when I found out. Then I go down a rabbit hole of how if that is true, then our relationship was never what I thought it was. When I get reminders of our memories together, it makes me sad. That initial twinge of sorrow is followed by resentment. I stop, thank God for her, and pray she is healthy and happy. I genuinely wish her well and then deliberately train my thoughts on other things. But recently, when the memories have come up, I've noticed a fondness occasionally creeping back in as I do *the work*. I lean into that! Life is too short for bitterness.

"He cuts off every branch in me that bears no fruit, while every branch that does bear fruit he prunes so that it will be even more fruitful." (John 15:2 NIV)

Can I also just say that I love Jesus, but I am not Jesus? I'm a hot mess of a flawed human being. I say bad words and frankly, cancer deserves some bad words. So, judge me all you want for the juxtaposition of my less-than-perfect ways mixed with Bible quotes. If you think that anyone who loves Jesus should be perfect, you're missing the whole point of the cross. I'm throwing that out there because I glean a lot of insight from scripture, but I find the world itself more palatable with four-letter words and an irreverent sense of humor. And once I was brave enough to embrace my true self unapologetically, I found out there are more people like me than I realized. I'm sorry it took me so long. I hope anyone reading this that may be offended by Jesus or four-letter words would look beyond that and glean some insight and/or comfort from my ordeal.

Meanwhile, in Boobland, there was boob drama everywhere. During that healing/waiting period, three boob incidents happened almost simultaneously in just my immediate family—many more in the friends, family of friends, and friends of friends realms. First, my beloved mother-in-law got scary results from a routine mammogram that required a biopsy. In the end, she was fine and quite healthy. Had it gone the other way, I would've been shaken to my core. She is quite disciplined in her eating and exercise routines and mostly the epitome of grounded composure. As I've said countless times, I am not in the camp of illness and disease being a stroke of bad luck, as much as western doctors claim otherwise. I believe there is always a factor, whether controllable and known by us or not.

Second, my eldest daughter finally had enough down time from college sports to get a much-needed boob reduction. She'd been wearing two sports bras at a time since she was about twelve just to contain *the girls*. She was getting it done and could hardly wait. And finally, my dear mother needed a lumpectomy for a highly suspicious mass on her breast that was *not* cancer, but the surgeon wanted it removed anyway for peace of mind. We have no genetic markers for breast cancer in my or my husband's family, so that is a ridiculous amount of boob drama for one family. And it seemed like we would all be having those surgeries within days of each other. Talk about triggering. My post-traumatic stress was off the charts. So, of course the patience gods—or whatever—said, "Let's up the ante."

On the way to my mom's pre-op appointment, I got a call from the rockstar's office canceling my surgery date (which they had just confirmed the day before). I was healed enough for the surgery to take place, finally! No more boob hole—but now, another setback! The last stitch of my patience must've slipped right out of the sunroof because I lost my shit.

In hindsight, this change allowed me to not only drive my mom to and from her surgery, but it also allowed me to fly to my daughter's house and stay with her for a week while she recovered. Despite the frustration of being put off yet again, I must admit the timing played out nicely. I was just so over the waiting. As I said, I was healed enough for them to book the surgery, and I just wanted the boob hole gone so I could look more like my normal self—especially now that I had started to feel like my normal self again. I just wanted to be done!

Chapter 9

Finding the Fix and a Nightmare Hospital Stay

I do not understand the mystery of grace;
only that it meets us where we are and doesn't
leave us where it found us.

~Anne Lamott

Finding out why things went so horribly wrong the first time and hoping to avoid the same fate with this flap, I'd seen a blood specialist, they ran labs, and I even did my own deep dives with my good friend, Google. I also jumped through hoops of red tape to get the renowned teaching hospital to give me my medical records. The more they gave me the run around, the more convinced I was that something big happened that no one was fessing up to—or, maybe they just didn't have their collective shit together. The third or fourth person I talked to in as many days finally apologized for the ridiculous runaround I'd gotten and dropped the medical records into my patient portal app. Easy peasy!

So it wasn't a big conspiracy. It was the "not having their shit together" thing. Phew!

My lab results came back unremarkable. The blood specialist found nothing that would indicate a bleeding issue resulting in a failed flap. Google gave me nothing but very low stats of these things occurring at all. When I was finally given the 3000+ pages of medical records (yes, 3000+ pages), I was basically looking for the needle in the haystack. Not to mention trying to understand medical jargon and abbreviations I'd not been trained to understand. Fun fact: every time a nurse or medical employee entered my room or interacted with me for any reason, it generated a medical record. To put it in perspective, remember: they checked for a doppler signal every hour for the first twenty-four, and then every two hours for the next forty-eight. When I finally found the actual surgery pages, they didn't say much except that I had bleeding, they couldn't stop it right away, and my IVs kept failing. And they said it in much more official wording, so I wasn't even sure I was reading it right.

I knew from previous procedures like blood draws that my veins were temperamental from having chemo. I'd declined the port because, frankly, having a hole in my chest sounded barbaric. And I told myself it was only four treatments, so my veins could handle it. Here is another example of wishing they'd just given me *all* the information, over-explained, and really painted the picture for me. Maybe it was a case of them not seeing the writing on the wall. Maybe it was one of those autopilot situations where they do this all day every day and forget that I don't. I can't say. All I know is that my veins became "like concrete" (their words) and since I only had the one arm to work with, that proved problematic during a fourteen-hour surgery. That explained all the abandoned IV sites I remembered seeing upon waking. My left arm is now forever off limits for BP, IVs, and anything that could cause a lymphedema risk—and had been since the first lymph node was removed. If I'd truly understood the whole picture, I'd have possibly decided the port was a better option to maintain the integrity of the veins in my right arm.

Twenty-four hours before this next surgery, I would get a peripherally inserted central catheter (PICC) line put in so there would be no issue with IVs. A PICC line is a thin, soft, long catheter that is inserted into a vein in your leg, arm, or neck. The tip of the catheter is positioned in a large vein that carries blood into the heart. It's used for long-term IV antibiotics or medications and blood draws. That was their big solution, and a big relief for me. Encouraging, anyway. Upon meeting with the rockstar and asking her what the hell happened, she sounded equally frustrated about how it all went. With her stellar reputation, I could understand. This was a big fat fail for the most part. I mean, two out of three flaps were good odds, but boobs are a package deal.

She dropped her stoic surgeon persona for a moment and said, exasperated, "Your veins are just bizarrely small. Hairlike!" She painted quite the picture with one sentence—and took her rockstar status up a notch for me. Microsurgery of hairlike veins. *Impressive!*

After the first surgery, I had standard post–flap surgery restrictions. No caffeine for weeks afterward, nothing that would constrict the blood vessels. No lifting, exercise, sweating, exertion. All the things. This time, it was driven home even more. No decaf either, which they let me have the first time. Basically, sit there until we tell you you're in the clear. And I did, not wanting to chance it. But again, with the nightmarish hospital stay—*man!* Some things just don't change. It was a shitshow. *Again!* I even recall, at one of my post-op appointments after this fix-it surgery, one of the nurse practitioners commiserating with me on this. She said it was ridiculous that they're a renowned hospital doing cutting-edge things that require delicate recoveries, yet putting their patients up in the oldest wing they've got.

"We're working on that," she assured me.

I don't even know what that means, and considering I'm not planning any more of these surgeries, I'm not sure I need to care. But my mind flashed back to all the chaos of tripping over each other and mad dashes to find working equipment or available equipment they needed.

But back to the surgery ...

Even when the rockstar told me I'd likely need one or two more surgeries to complete everything, I maintained my calm going into the surgery. That news wanted to fling me over the edge, but I held my ground steadily. One flap, one four- to five-hour surgery, and another four- to five-day hospital stay. I had this. That fix-it surgery went much better than the last two, but the post-surgery experience was par for the course with the same "old" wing and almost the same room, the same hourly doppler checks, the same panic-inducing BAIR hugger, and the same uncomfortable beds that have obviously been around for a long time (because they dipped so severely in the middle, crawling out of bed became quite literal). There were a couple new additions though, including two different roommates from hell—one from South Hell. There was also a lesser restriction on visitors, so I got my husband for large portions of the days, as well as a couple other visitors. I guess it was a tradeoff, because it certainly helped diffuse the crazy of the roommates.

First up, the roommate from South Hell.

I never got a look at her, but I heard her well enough. Everyone did. She sounded older—or at least older than me. She was clearly an adult, but beyond being reasoned with. Each hour when the nurses came in to check the doppler signal, this chick would flip out—every single time, without fail. It went something like this:

"Ugh!"

"Oh my God!"

"Not again."

"Stop it!"

"Turn it down."

It was a variation of some or all of that on repeat. Every time! And it wasn't an "under your breath" kind of complaint. Instead, she competed with the volume of doppler. The first few times I heard the nurses trying to explain it to her. When that didn't help, I guess they stopped bothering. Did I mention this happened every hour? I'm not sure if they moved her or if she was discharged, but that only lasted a day. Even the people pleaser in me ran out of the benefit of the doubt to give this lady. It set my nerves on edge, more than they already were. So much for not raising the heart rate. And I'm not *hating* on the roommate. On the contrary, reflecting my irreverent sense of humor, I asked the nurses if they thought there was a hidden camera somewhere. I mean, her reaction really was a surreal and ridiculous level of absurdity.

Roommate number two was much quieter, sort of. By the time she moved in, I was able to get up and go to the bathroom by myself, so I saw her. She was the cutest, sweetest looking older woman. She had thick glasses and a full face of makeup—like, vaudeville style—and the sweetest smile. She didn't talk; she had a trach. This trach gurgled around the clock, though, and made me do the quick swallow thing you do when you were trying not to vomit. And it had to be cleaned out regularly, which produced a whole new level of gurgling sounds. I may suffer from a bit of misophonia, which in simple terms is a strong aversion to noises, specifically mouth noises. My beloved twelve-year-old dog can send me over the edge in 2.3 seconds with her constant licking noises. This neighbor's noises didn't exactly send me over the edge—it just grossed me out. She was so sweet I just wanted to hug her. While the sounds were next-level disgusting, I found myself calmly and earnestly praying for her instead of getting annoyed. I overheard doctors tell her at one point that the trach would be the resolution to her issue, with no further treatment of radiation or chemo required. I gathered that meant she'd had cancer. I said a prayer of gratitude for her *good* news and thanked God for my own circumstances, which, despite my issues, I would not trade for hers. Again, recognizing that perspective is an invaluable gift. But (yep, there's a "but") …

She was apparently a night owl and slept all day. This meant she left her light on all night, which shone down perfectly on me. All night long, every damn night! No joke. It was like a spotlight. I felt like I should be on stage with a gold statue, thanking the Academy, instead of lying in a hospital bed. And she liked to listen to some old school talk radio thing. I'm guessing earbuds are before her time. On one special night, her husband stayed later than usual and decided to answer a spam call on his cell phone and argue with the guy—out loud, for a long time. My husband happened to be there at the time, and I had to talk him off the ledge of *taking the guy out*. Okay, not literally. But for my husband to even be triggered by someone to that degree speaks volumes. His fuse is longer than anyone's I've ever met, by at least double. I'm quite sure that's why we have such a successful marriage, but I digress. Suffice it to say, it was annoying.

By the last night in hospital hell, the fourth one, I couldn't take it any longer. I felt like I was losing my mind. My nerves were fried. It wasn't just the neighbors; it was everything. Did I forget to mention that I got hives *again*? Despite troubleshooting the reason in hopes of avoiding them this time around, there they were—but only at the incision/surgery sites, this time. I'm still not 100 percent sure what caused them. Maybe I'll never have another surgery and it won't matter. My words to God's ears.

For four days, I could only sleep in fragments. I was constantly performing my therapy tricks to avoid the anxiety and panic. By the fifth morning, I was all over anyone in scrubs like white on rice about getting discharged. The original paperwork said five days max, and I was holding them to it. Once they greenlit my discharge, it still took them six hours to get their ducks in a row and release me. I spent much of those six hours pacing the halls like a caged animal. Some might wonder why I didn't just leave. Well, hospitals are savvy to that. They leave every IV, bandage, and piece of tape in place until you get your walking papers. Believe me when I say I wanted to let the professionals untangle me from my leash of tubes, tape, and bullshit. It was just too much. It's not like the movies, where the pretty patient rips all their stuff off and leaves. I tried to rest while I waited, but within minutes I would be up pacing like the caged animal again. Fun fact about discharge protocol is that once they agree to discharge you, they no longer administer medication. So while they take hours to release you, they apparently will not give you anything to help you with pain or to chill you the fuck out while you wait. But at least I was feeling good enough after this surgery to pace unassisted. I'll take that win.

After three days of being back in my own bed with my own things—and the blessed peace and quiet—I still couldn't sleep for more than an hour at a time. By the fourth day at home, I would sit and sob that I just wanted to sleep. Yeah, surgery-induced insomnia is a thing! I couldn't make sense of it, so I started searching for answers. Thank you, Google:

> "Insomnia after surgery is common. There are many potential causes, including pain, medications, anxiety, and the unfamiliar environment of a hospital. Typically, symptoms last a few days to a few weeks. Major surgeries tend to disrupt sleep more than minor procedures." (www.medicalnewstoday.com)

This is where my love of books is key. Since I was a kid, I could easily blow off bedtime for the sake of a good plot, and I had a new series I'd saved just for this recovery. Thanks to the insomnia, I blew through them in five days. They were everything I needed: long, consuming, dramatic, transporting, tragic, page-turning, and a can't-put-down guilty pleasure. And as usual, the book was better than the movie. Way better. But I did have the movie versions to binge after I finished the books. Shout out to Anna Todd for the *After* series. Love it or hate it, I for one will always think of these stories fondly for getting me through.

When I finally did start sleeping, I began to feel like myself again. But as things healed and settled, I realized that more surgery was definitely in my future. The thing about one *normal* flap with *normal* fat is that it did not look like a flap made with omentum. Once a concave hole, the omentum flap was noticeably bigger than the other one. At my three-month post op, I began asking about the next and hopefully final surgery. They told me they were booking into April of the following year. Almost another year of waiting. I took it in stride—not my first rodeo. But the good news is that when this one finally happened, it would be an outpatient procedure. No hospital stay! I'd already become accustomed to the absolute chaos of a rockstar's schedule, so I took the win and called it a day.

I know! I hear you all asking: *why is the chick still going so hard for the boobs?* But hang with me. But we're almost there! I've been swimming through this dark tunnel and holding my breath for so long, but I'm almost to the surface. I can see the sunlight shining down into the water. I can see the end. If I just hold my breath a little longer and keep swimming, I'll break through the surface and be free. Then I can dry out, bask in the sun, and put all this behind me. I will get to buy *and wear* bras for the first time in years. Yeah, I know—most women are like, *you must be joking. I'd love to not wear a bra.* But let me paint this picture: I've had to wear soft sleep-type bras for gentle support, soft cami-type tops on top of that to tuck in, so that the sensitive scars on my abdomen don't get irritated by my jeans, pants, seams, etc. and then wear a regular top over that. For *years!* And the trial, error, and expense of all that is exhausting. I was mostly looking forward to being able to just throw on some clothes and not have to overthink it—and maybe ditch a few layers while I'm at it. The bonus would be not feeling self-conscious to the point of anxiety anymore, and just living my life.

But not so fast ...

Chapter 10

The Final Surgery, Finally (Thank God for Hernias and Outpatient)

Sometimes you win, sometimes you lose,
sometimes it rains.
~Ron Shelton, *Bull Durham*

Throughout the years of waiting between surgeries, it's important to remember we'd gone through a pandemic and a complete shutdown of the world as we knew it. And while things have largely gotten back to *normal*, most of this went down when things were far from it.

In the name of staying healthy, I'd quit going to church and instead streamed services online. I would mortifyingly ask if my friends were relatively healthy before agreeing to attend small gatherings. I didn't fly unless necessary and unavoidable—like to see my kids. When I did hit the *fuck it* button and go somewhere extremely public, I used every tool in my toolbox to dial down the worry and panic. Before you let all the opinions fly, I wasn't scared of getting sick. I feared getting sick *and* it resulting in the medical world canceling my surgeries. Testing for cooties forty-eight hours before surgeries was the norm for two of the four surgeries I had. The third one happened when things started relaxing again. By the fourth, we were back to business as usual. Mostly. There were a few times we'd have friends over and a couple of them would show up clearly recovering from some cootie and I'd work my way through the panic, hugs hello and goodbye, etc. It was a shitty way to live. Judge away, but you don't know if you don't know. I promise not to judge you for that. The times I threw caution to the wind were trips to sunny places with the promise of endless amounts of vitamin D and healing negative ions. I even took two of those trips with the boob hole, with lots of boob pad options to even out the chest and look normal(ish) in a swimsuit—even if I didn't feel normal.

The thing about easing up on my crowd anxiety is that I began to ease up on everything. It's easy to forget and go on autopilot. The more normal things I did, the more normal I felt. I would sometimes forget who I was now—the chick with no core strength or solid muscle tone; which is likely how I threw my back out and possibly gave myself a hernia somewhere between the third and fourth surgeries. The thing about going from surgery to surgery is that there wasn't any real time to get my strength back. And I didn't do anything extreme, just moved some books around one day. My back began having small spasms that night which worsened each day, until I ended up in the ER a few days before we were set to travel to one of those sunny places. Some muscle relaxers and bed rest got me feeling well enough to get excited about our tropical vacation. It was mid-February and I couldn't wait to be warm. I had two normal-ish boobs this time. The flight went well, and it wasn't long before we touched down in the land of the sun. I even got a kick out of watching the guy across the aisle from me sanitize every space he'd be touching over the course of the flight. I was finally not so worried about cooties.

It had been a minute since I'd run around half naked. I no longer felt as self-conscious about my boobs, so I was happy to don a swimsuit. That's when I noticed a lump in my abdomen just above my newly constructed navel. Having a life-threatening disease *twice* and some nightmarish surgeries can make one over-analyze every weird ache, pain, and lump. Everyone on our trip seemed to think it was nothing, so I went with that and mostly put it out of my mind. Upon arriving home, two things happened: I got the airplane cooties I'd been so diligent to avoid for two years, and the lump had grown. I no longer internally mocked the guy overly cleaning his airplane space, and wished I'd been more like him. I was kicking myself for not maniacally sanitizing my own space. While I wasn't flipping out per se about a weird lump (not my first rodeo), I was absolutely gearing up for the self-advocacy parade I knew was coming.

They were tentatively scheduling this outpatient (hopefully last) surgery for April, as I said. It was late February. I conveniently had a routine ultrasound and appointment with my oncologist coming up and asked if she'd be willing to capture a shot of the lump while I was there. I knew the plastic surgeon would want me to get one. My oncologist accommodated, with almost no advocating from me. Maybe the tides were turning. The oncologist confirmed that the lump looked like a possible hernia (umbilical, she said) but admitted it was not her area of expertise.

I began sending photos and messages to my team of plastic surgeons and nurses, along with the results of the ultrasound from my oncologist's hospital. My rockstar surgeon was out the country doing rockstar shit and so were her best helpers, who were also *my* best helpers, except for one who'd just come back from maternity leave. She was the first to respond and wanted to see me right away. At the end of February, the scheduler began calling to set me up for that April surgery. This scheduler is a saint, by the way. She's been working with the rockstar at least as long as I have. She's had to call me more than once to reschedule me, usually at the last minute. She's heard me cry, lose my shit, and use most of the four-letter words I know, yet she has maintained her professionalism. I am in awe of her. I even got to meet her face to face once at a post-op appointment from the previous surgery.

She had to get some information from me and came into my room after the appointment. As soon as I heard her voice, I knew exactly who she was. I'd prayed on more than one occasion for an opportunity to have a candid conversation with her where I could apologize for *all the emotions*. I took a deep breath and began my sincere apology. I told her how sorry I was for *always* losing my shit on her. I might've even used those exact words. I don't actually like behaving like an asshole, I just have some deep-seated self-control issues I'm working on. She was the epitome of grace and might've even got a tear in her eye that someone acknowledged how much shit she undoubtedly puts up with. I mean, I know I'm not the only one getting rescheduled. And also, how cool is it that I got the opportunity to do that? I thanked God repeatedly on my way out. But I digress. When the scheduler called me for this next surgery, I explained about the hernia (that I didn't actually know I had yet, but suspected). I told her I was hoping to only go under general anesthesia once more and that I wanted the hernia repair along with the boob fix. If this sounds weirdly like I was ordering lunch in a restaurant, I agree. I very matter-of-factly told her how I wanted this to go down. I've found that the medical professionals I've dealt with seem to appreciate and respond well to that. I'll spare you that rabbit hole of reasoning, but I've pondered *the why* a time or two. The scheduler said she'd let the team know and start working on it.

Once the nurse practitioner saw the photos in my chart, she confirmed right away that she suspected a hernia. She explained that she used to diagnose and repair them in infants before switching to plastics. When I saw her in person a few days later, she said it wasn't umbilical but incisional. I thought, *Incisional, meaning it's from the surgery?* And she agreed it was not only reasonable to want only one surgery, but it should also absolutely go down that way. *Great!* I just needed the rockstar on board. The NP also said I'd need to get the general surgeon on board who harvested the omentum and basically created the incision that led to the hernia to begin with. And that if that general surgeon couldn't repair it, the rockstar "would just do it."

It is not lost on me that I was now charged with doing the legwork to coordinate some major moving parts of my own surgery. But in my single mindedness, I kept my eye on the prize. One surgery, two fixes, no waiting. I called the general surgeon right away. It turned out the general didn't do hernia repairs. *Good!* Simpler to schedule, to my way of thinking. But it did cross my mind that this surgeon could readily help create an environment that could cause a hernia but did not perform surgeries that would repair one if it happened. I mean, I'm a relatively intelligent person with a fair amount of common sense. Just make it make sense to me. But again, I had bigger fish to fry. As I said, it seemed like it would make things much simpler. I told the rockstar's NP and the scheduler right away that the general surgeon was out. They still had the surgery happening at the beginning of April, unless there was a cancellation beforehand. If I wanted to be on the cancellation list, I'd have to give up my April surgery date. And I wasn't guaranteed a sooner date–it could end up being later, even. *Huh?!* Again, just make it make sense. I decided not to *roll the dice.* I took to wearing compression camis and belly bands to hopefully keep things stable until then.

But I had a couple of life things happening in the meantime. One of my closest friend's daughters (my eldest daughter's best friend) was getting married in mid-March, and right after that my husband was taking me along on a work trip to San Diego, where he would golf Torrey Pines for the first time and I'd get to play the pampered wife for a couple days at the resort. One dressy, dancing event and one swimsuit event with the hernia lump. Both once-in-a-lifetime events that I didn't want to miss. But I equally did not want to *anger* the hernia.

I can't explain it, but I just knew in my bones that one or both of those things were going to get derailed over this surgery. It's how my experiences with the rockstar seemed to go. Some of the most devout manifesters may say I willed it. I disagree. I prayed it wouldn't and planned as if both were going to happen for me. I still have a couple outfits hanging in my closet with the tags on for that San Diego trip I never took. I did get to attend the wedding though. Thank God! Clearly the more important of two, if one had to go. Missing that would've seriously pissed me off. But the scheduler did call the day before the wedding, while we were decorating the hall, to tell me the date had changed again. *Shocker!*

Let me back up for a minute. She had already called two days prior to tell me they were working on a closer date, but the days they wanted were no longer available—not even the original date in April. *I guess she gave up my original date after all.* She said it with a lot more words and reasoning, but it doesn't even matter. Dates kept changing, subsequently changing everything in their paths. Available ORs were apparently the issue and *if I could just be patient.* I calmly told her that I could be as patient as they needed me to be, after all *we'd* been through.

"But if someone could just let the hernia know that's what we're doing," I added, "that'd be great."

God bless this woman. She not only laughed, but also said, "Yeah if we could just get the hernia to chill the fuck out."

Then she stopped mid-sentence like, *what did I just say?* I laughed out loud at her response and thanked her for saying it.

She began apologizing and said, jokingly, "Please don't tell my boss."

I told her that not only would I not be *telling on her*, but that she'd just earned my lifelong respect for being on my level in that moment. So, at that point we had *no* date for surgery and a hernia with a mind of its own.

I was beyond frustrated after that call. Relaying the story to my niece (and hairdresser) at my hair appointment that afternoon, she immediately insisted I *had* to send an email of complaint. She pleaded with me to just put it in writing "in case something serious happens because of the schedule changes." I wanted to send it. I did! But I struggled with my inner *Karen*. I really don't like to let her out of the closet I keep her locked in. I tend to drag my filter around kicking and screaming as it is, so being confrontational without coming off as an asshole can be a challenge for me. That day, I proved to myself that I can say hard things with finesse. It also turns out that email got me fast tracked. *Thank you, Niece, for the push!*

The picture I included with my long ranting message to the NP that afternoon showed that the hernia was indeed getting worse by the day despite my efforts to keep it contained. It gave no fucks about the rockstar's timeline or the OR schedules. I copied the rockstar on it. I specifically addressed this barrage of pre-op videos I was sent, detailing my upcoming procedure, post op care, flowery marketing clips from the hospital's team of surgeons, and the *known* risks—one of which was hernias, that I had to sign off on that I'd watched and understood. By the way, this is the first time I'd ever been sent required videos pre-surgery, and if you're counting, this would be my fourth with this team.

This was my message, which I edited down from an incredibly thorough rant (because there's a word limit for messages in the health chart app):

I received/viewed all the required pre-op videos today. Thanks for sending. They were quite informative. Especially the part about my reconstruction being a hernia risk. I've been in this reconstruction with you for years now and this is the first I've heard of a known risk of hernias. Had I known, I may have opted for an alternative. It's a moot point now but it would've been nice to know prior to beginning. And I just got a call from the scheduler saying my surgery date is not confirmed at all now, changed from yesterday. I appreciate all the moving parts required to make these surgeries happen, but this whole experience has been one thing after another. From the very start, nothing has gone smoothly or as planned. I'm trying to take it in stride, but this is my body and my life, and both seem to get more compromised with each procedure. The videos go on and on about how you want to give patients their life back. So far, this has not been my experience. Respectfully, Carol

They called in the late afternoon Friday as we were setting up for the wedding and told me I'd be having surgery Monday. *In three days!* Just wow. And I'd love to tell you that this was the first time I'd be jumping through hoops to get another surgery under my belt in a rush. It wasn't, but it was the first time for *this* much of a rush. Anesthesia called for a video visit; there was no time for an in-person appointment. I had to get the pre-op wash at the drug store over the weekend instead of from the doctor. And of course, there would be no time for a PICC line insertion. Those have to happen 24 hours prior to surgery and they didn't do them on weekends. But it was outpatient and therefore quick. The need for extra IVs was low. I tried not to *enjoy myself* too much at the wedding, but let me tell you, if anyone deserved a drink, it was me.

"It's the last surgery," I kept telling myself. *Eye on the prize! And it's outpatient! Short and sweet! No nightmare hospital stay!*

On surgery day, I had all the nerves. When you arrive at the end of a very long, nightmarish tunnel and see the light, sometimes it's hard to trust it's not a train. After all the ups and downs, starts and stops, I couldn't quite believe I was finally at the end. Almost. When the rockstar popped in to draw on me, I made sure to point out every little thing that might need tucking or otherwise fine tuning. She happily accommodated and even added her own little areas she wanted to perfect. Fine by me! It gave me a moment of exhale that she was being meticulous and ... final?! But I couldn't completely relax. For whatever reason—maybe because of the sheer chaos leading up to this one—I struggled with the doom mentality. At one point, I even told my husband that I wanted him to tell my eldest (who is my extremely cautious, ever prudent daughter) to let her guard down more in life and especially in love. He told me to shut up and tell her myself later. That might be a direct quote.

I'm relieved I kept my guard up as they wheeled me into the OR. The anesthesiologist was going over his procedure with me while nurses buzzed around me, doing what they do. One approached me to place the BP band on my arm. When she went to the left side, I had to stop her and remind her it can only go on the right arm. I even had the bracelet on to alert them. What if I'd been sedated already? Seriously?! What the hell, people? C'mon! My heart races just typing it. Once they got me all hooked up, they told me I needed to take some deep breaths because my blood pressure was up. *No shit! A little nervous here that you degreed medical professionals might actually fuck this up while I'm unconscious. But yeah, I'll take some deep breaths for you, Judy.*

I woke up after a quick two-and-a-half hour nap feeling better than I thought possible. I kept waiting for the *suck* to hit me and it just didn't. Comparatively speaking, this was a walk in the park from top to bottom. Speaking of walking, I did, every day, from day one. And at six weeks post-op to the day, I was back to the gym—treadmill only, to start. I was determined to get my core strength back and never subject myself to a hernia again. One drag of this recovery was having to wear a belly band twenty-four/seven for six months post op. I got them down to just during the day after three months.

"Especially while doing activities," they warned.

I wasn't trying to risk it. If they'd insisted on twenty-four/seven, I would do it. Six months for a lifetime of normal? Done! When I finally got to see

Dr. Rockstar in person, shortly after the three-month mark, she concurred that the belly band as needed was safe enough. She added that as long as I didn't see any dramatic weight changes, my breasts would continue to look ... *done*. Hallelujah! *For the love of God, can I be done having surgeries? Pretty please with a cherry on top?!*

I wish I could tell you that I was done with all the medical stuff and got to go live my life with cancer completely in the rearview. I wish I could tell you that yearly scans didn't still unnerve me, or that I still don't overthink the food I eat, the products I use, and the things I overthink about. I recently had my yearly breast MRI and will have my follow-up appointment with my oncologist. I'm happy to have a team of doctors making sure I stay cancer free. So, I trade my dread of these appointments for gratefulness that I have so many eyes on me making sure I stay healthy. This is where having a routine comes in handy. This is where journaling, positive affirmations, prayer, exercise, actively seeking peace, and even incessant label reading help to calm my fear. Some of my non-negotiables are clean eating and quality products for my skin and in my household. I hear all the time, "but it's so expensive." And I agree. It is undeniably more expensive than the products that readily line the shelves of every retail establishment, but it is not as expensive as surgery, chemotherapy, radiation, and funerals. Read that again!

When I get asked about my experience, I see people's eyes begin to glaze over with the sheer amount of information I spew at them. I've learned to tone it down a bit. I'm just so passionate about avoiding cancer and helping others do the same. What I say now is that I've been on this journey for more than a decade—thirteen years and counting. And it all started with just one change. What if you changed just one thing this month to better your health? And then did it again next month? By the end of the year, that would be twelve things you've changed to improve your quality of life. That's 156 things I'd have changed in thirteen years. I'd guess that number is a lot higher for me but I like I said, I can be a dog with bone. And for the love of God, do not beat yourself up for what you *haven't* changed. Just take the first step, or the next step, and then another. And then ...

Chapter 11

Still Grateful, Especially for the Rearview Mirror

Forgive yourself for not knowing what you didn't know before you learned it.
~Maya Angelou

I started writing all this down when I realized what a shitshow it had become, and how it could benefit someone else to know the hell I went through. I truly didn't envision a second book on this cancer journey of mine. One of my repeated thoughts is, "why go through something like this, if you can't use it to help the next guy with all the things you've learned along the way?" What's the point? I've heard in church a lot that God doesn't waste a hurt. I guess that's what I'm doing. Not wasting a hurt. And while this book may land for some as a giant list of complaints, I want to assure you that the gift of perspective is not lost on me. I got to a healthy enough place after cancer to undergo breast reconstruction. I have lain next to patients in hospitals who made me thankful for *my* shitshow instead of theirs. I've found grace for myself and others along the way. I have a second act dream job as a writer and author that allows me to share my experience and maybe help someone else in the process. The list goes on ...

I've met plenty of women who decided to forego any kind of reconstructive surgery. I've also met plenty who decided to forego any traditional, toxic treatments. The biggest thing I hope anyone going through cancer can take away from this is that there is no cookie-cutter solution. As undeniably unique as we all are, so are our paths, solutions, and remedies. And while sharing our experiences can undoubtedly make us feel less alone, my path may not be yours.

My biggest non-negotiable for anyone facing something like cancer, or any health crisis, is to advocate for yourself. Be the squeaky wheel, the pain in the ass, if that's what it takes to get you the care and end result you're looking for—although I highly recommend muzzling your inner Karen whenever possible. My husband is always telling me it's not what I say, but how I say it.

He'd say, "Babe, you come in at a ten and then have nowhere left to go. You've got to start at like a three and slowly escalate if needed. You can't jump right to setting people on fire."

Noted! Like my grandma always said, "You get more bees with honey."

Another non-negotiable I've decided for myself is getting good sleep. I take magnesium every night and keep my room dark and cool. Mostly, I listen to my body. I pay attention to my nervous system. I do not *power through* stressful situations; I remove myself. When things feel overwhelming, I recognize it as my body's response to trauma. And instead of letting my system power through and store that as the appropriate response to overwhelm, I let my system know that's not *how we roll.* Not anymore.

I've proven to myself that I can face the hard things, the infuriating things, with a kind heart and non-bitchy tone, while also not taking any shit. It may not be my default setting or what comes naturally to me, but it feels more comfortable everyday. And one day, it may feel like my default setting. Also, I've found some pretty sweet bees with my hard-earned honey. I even feel a tremendous amount of peace about those relationships I've left behind. I view all my relationships through a different lens, now. I've realized that if old relationships aren't evolving with me, they will hinder (and likely are already hindering) my growth—and probably theirs too. I've adopted a more chill approach of not forcing things and walking away from chaos. Full disclosure: I'm pretty good at it except where my kids are concerned. I'm still navigating the "mom of adult children" thing. I can't help my *buttinsky* nature where they are concerned, much to their annoyance. But our rich, highly entertaining conversations more than make up for my over-*momming.* I hope so, anyway.

The thing about writers, or most of the ones I know, is that we love lessons in the form of stories, and I've always got a story for my kids to go with the lesson. Some people might see my storytelling as a way of making it *all about me.* I can assure you that is not my heart—it's just my way of trying to relate to others, to truly put myself in their shoes and say *I feel you, and I hope that makes you feel less alone.* Isn't that the whole point anyway? To feel a connectedness to each other? Otherwise, what is the point? So, my quest going forward is to seek out and nurture my mutually connected relationships and grow—with two boobs, a calm immune system, and a bonus flat-ish belly. And to leave the *rockstars* behind me for good, as much as I'm grateful to them for their incredible talent, efforts, and the boobs they brought me. If I'm ever in places where I feel like I need to *earn* affection, I find a new place. And I continue to work out my issues so they don't get stuck in my tissues.

Each of us going through a medical crisis must decide what's important for ourselves and what we're willing to do to get it. Whether that is modifications to diet, lifestyle, relationships, or all of the above. I still think boobs are overrated, but I'm extremely happy to have a matching set ... *ish*. It helps that Barbie made no nipples cool again. And never having to worry about *headlights* makes getting dressed everyday even more of a no brainer. Life is short. I'd rather spend it living than overthinking, which a cancer crisis can certainly cause one to do. I choose my words, my thoughts, and how I spend my time carefully these days. Like I said, I wouldn't wish cancer on anyone, but the perspective from this side is nice. I've made so many mistakes throughout my life, but I no longer hold myself or any-one else to a ridiculous standard of perfection in the hope of being good enough to receive love. I hope I've modeled that for my children and that they will always know they are enough, exactly as they are. I hope those no longer in my life are abundantly happy, healthy, and living well.

I am so grateful to the rockstar and her team, despite the chaos. She gave me the "all clear" to go live my life—within reason, of course, as I am still healing and will hold certain risks now (such as hernias) due to my new physical dynamics. But I am blissfully wearing swimsuits and feeling like myself again ... *ish*. I'm not cuing the hallelujah choir just yet.

I've recently resumed seeing my naturopathic doctor to finalize *Project: Take My Life Back*. I hadn't seen her in almost two years, with all the surgery/recovery drama. Now that I had my *walking papers* from the surgeon, I wanted to revisit my health regimen of supplements, medication, and anything else that would help me bounce back. I had this lingering fatigue that kept derailing my attempts. I assumed it was my body needing time to heal from all it had been through. I reject the narrative I repeatedly hear from people my age that I was just getting old. Older, yes. Not old! One thing naturopaths do that western medicine does not is get extremely extensive blood tests. My recent lab results showed I tested positive for the Epstein Barr virus that was wreaking havoc on my immune system, nervous system, joints, and general disposition. It's highly contagious, and one way to get it is via blood transfusion. I was shocked, but not. As the *why* girl, I could obsess if that's how I got it in the first place. It would definitely explain the chronic fatigue over the past couple years. But I've got to focus on the bigger fish. Getting over the virus is the priority. I'm currently on my squeaky hamster wheel of research and advocating for myself again—still?! I feel fortunate that I can see a naturopathic doctor to pursue alternative treatments. Again, these types of doctors are not covered by insurance and can be extremely expensive. But they can offer some of the best non-toxic ways to heal our bodies, like vitamin C infusions and hyperbaric oxygen chambers, to name a couple. I'm hoping, praying, and trusting that I can and will find my way back to a *normal* level of good health and energy. It's a process, but I'm here for it, figuratively and literally. And for that, I can cue the hallelujah choir.

For more on this, head to www.wylliegirl.com and download a free bonus chapter and my cheat sheet of tips and tricks as a thank you from me.

Thanks for walking through this journey with me.

Wishing you all good health, a good life, and good books.

Acknowledgments

My deepest gratitude first and foremost is for God and His mighty plan. Thank you for showing me that even the messiest of humans have something beautiful to offer.

Thank you to my ridiculously cool family. You all are proof that God loves me and wants me to be happy.

My husband, Rob, is truly the love of my life and my favorite person on the planet. His quiet support and irreverent humor lift me up in more ways than I can even explain. And while he is not a book guy, he promised to read every word I ever write. Thanks for recognizing zoning out and staring off into space is sometimes me working.

My two daughters, Madison and Alyssa, make me want to be the best version of myself. I am in awe of the humans I got to help create and raise into the confident, kind, hard-working, Jesus-loving young women you are. I learn from you every day, and I'm so grateful I get to be your momma.

To my inner circle—you know who you are. Thanks for believing in me and telling me I could do it, even when I didn't always believe it ... and for the cheap (free) therapy sessions, too. You're more important to me than you'll ever know, though I do try to show you as often as I can.

About the Author

Carol is a retired stay-at-home mom-turned-bestselling author. She lives on an olive orchard in rural Northern California with her husband, two dogs, and two cats. In her debut nonfiction bestseller, *Chemo Pissed Me Off*, Carol offers real insight for anyone facing cancer, illness, or any of life's challenges. She is humorous and sometimes irreverent while showing us how to take something as ominous as cancer and turn it into an opportunity for growth. Now a full-time author, she has published a series of children's books and her new nonfiction follow up to *Chemo Pissed Me Off, Boobs Are Overrated*. Carol plans to continue to write and publish books in multiple genres. She hopes to inspire others by transparently sharing her experiences through her writing.

NOW IT'S YOUR TURN

Discover the EXACT three-step
blueprint you need to become
a bestselling author in as little as three months.

Self-Publishing School helped me,
and now I want them to help
you with this FREE resource to
begin outlining your book!

Even if you're busy, bad at writing,
or don't know where to start,
you CAN write a bestseller and build your best life.

With tools and experience across a
variety of niches and professions,
Self-Publishing School is the only resource you need to
take your book to the finish line!

DON'T WAIT

Say "YES" to becoming a bestseller:

https://self-publishingschool.com/friend/
Follow the steps on the page to get a FREE
resource to get started on your book and unlock a
discount to get started with selfpublishing.com.

I HAVE A FREE GIFT FOR YOU!

Visit my website to download your cheat sheet of tips and tricks now as a thank you for reading my book.

Made in the USA
Las Vegas, NV
19 November 2024

12152464R00089